PANDEMICS

WHAT EVERYONE NEEDS TO KNOW

PETER C. DOHERTY

D0067658

OXFORD
UNIVERSITY PRESS

OXFORD
UNIVERSITY PRESS

Oxford University Press is a department of the University of Oxford.
It furthers the University's objective of excellence in research, scholarship,
and education by publishing worldwide.

Oxford   New York
Auckland   Cape Town   Dar es Salaam   Hong Kong   Karachi
Kuala Lumpur   Madrid   Melbourne   Mexico City   Nairobi
New Delhi   Shanghai   Taipei   Toronto

With offices in
Argentina   Austria   Brazil   Chile   Czech Republic   France   Greece
Guatemala   Hungary   Italy   Japan   Poland   Portugal   Singapore
South Korea   Switzerland   Thailand   Turkey   Ukraine   Vietnam

Oxford is a registered trademark of Oxford University Press
in the UK and certain other countries.

Published in the United States of America by
Oxford University Press
198 Madison Avenue, New York, NY 10016

© Peter C. Doherty 2013

Library of Congress Cataloging-in-Publication Data

Doherty, P. C. (Peter C.)
Pandemics / Peter C. Doherty.
p. ; cm.—(What everyone needs to know)
Includes bibliographical references.
Summary: "From HIV to H1N1, pandemics pose one of the greatest threats to global
health in the twenty-first century. Defined as epidemics of infectious disease across
large geographic areas, pandemics can disseminate globally with incredible speed as
humans and goods move faster than ever before. While restricted travel, quarantine,
vaccines, drugs, and education can reduce the severity of many outbreaks, factors such
as global warming, population density, and antibiotic resistance will complicate our
ability to fight disease. Respiratory infections like influenza and SARS spread quickly
as a consequence of modern, mass air travel, while unsafe health practices promote the
spread of viruses like HIV/AIDS and hepatitis C. In Pandemics: What Everyone Needs
to Know, Nobel Prize-winning immunologist Peter Doherty addresses the history
of pandemics and the ones that persist today, what promotes global spread, types of
pathogens and the level of threat they pose, as well as how to combat outbreaks and
mitigate their effects"—Provided by publisher.
ISBN 978–0–19–989812–1 (pbk. : alk. paper) — ISBN 978–0–19–989810–7
(cloth : alk. paper)
I. Title.   II. Series: What everyone needs to know.
[DNLM: 1. Pandemics—history.   2. Pandemics—prevention & control.
3. Disaster Planning.   4. World Health. WA 105]
RA399.5
362.1028′9—dc23
2013004528

1 3 5 7 9 8 6 4 2
Printed in the United States of America
on acid-free paper

The deviation of man from the state in which he was originally placed by nature seems to have proved to him a prolific source of diseases.

—*Edward Jenner (1749–1823), pioneer of the smallpox vaccine, sometimes called the "father of immunology"*

TABLE OF CONTENTS

ACKNOWLEDGMENTS   xiii

ABBREVIATIONS   xv

INTRODUCTION   xxi

1   Infection and Immunity   1

What is the difference between a virus and a bacterium?   2

What is the difference between RNA and DNA?   9

Aren't viruses also much smaller than bacteria?   13

Why is it important to distinguish viruses from bacteria when discussing pandemics?   15

Are colds and flu caused by hundreds of viruses?   17

What exactly is a pathogen?   19

How does infection happen?   22

What is snot?   26

What is a horizontal infection? Is there another kind?   26

Are all virus and bacterial infections bad for us?   27

If there is a bacterial and protozoal "microbiome," is there also a "virome"?   28

What does "immunity" mean?   30

What are monoclonal antibodies?   37

Would you describe mAbs as drugs or vaccines?   39

What are vaccines?   40

2   Pandemics, Epidemics, and Outbreaks   42

What is the exact definition of pandemic?   42

Who declares a pandemic?   43

Was the H1N1 "swine flu" really so mild?   44

How does the WHO operate?   45

Should the pandemic classification system be refined?   48

How does a pandemic differ from an epidemic or an outbreak?   49

Do all pandemics involve infection?   51

What does the term "zoonosis" mean?   52

*What is an endemic infection, and how does it differ from an epidemic
infection?*   54

Are plants also included in the world of pandemics?   55

In Summary   55

3   The SARS Warning   56

Why was SARS so scary?   56

How did SARS spread so quickly through hospitals?   57

What caused SARS and where did the pathogen come from?   59

*Aside from "natural" reservoirs, are there other potential
sources of SARS?*   61

What steps were taken to stop the SARS outbreak?   61

*Did the SARS experience have long-term effects, and what lessons
were learned?*   63

4   Tuberculosis and Influenza   66

Why should TB and influenza be considered together?   66

What is the current situation with TB?   66

Is multi-drug-resistant TB still an issue?   68

What is being done to combat the MDR TB threat?   70

Why might influenza remain the most obvious known pandemic threat?   70

What are the different kinds of influenza viruses?   72

What is antigenic shift and why is it so dangerous?   74

Are birds and pigs our main concern when it comes to catching the flu?   78

What was so special about the virus that caused the 1918–1919 influenza pandemic?   79

Is our capacity to counter influenza improving?   82

Are we making progress with flu vaccines?   83

Apart from vaccines, are there other products available to prevent infection?   86

How afraid should we be of influenza?   88

5   Fledermaus to Field Mouse   90

What's a fledermaus?   90

Is it unusual that fruit bats carry SARS?   90

Are the henipaviruses potential pandemic pathogens?   93

Is Ebola the scariest of all viruses?   94

What exactly is a hemorrhagic disease?   96

Are filoviruses the main cause of hemorrhagic fevers?   98

6   Virus Vectors   102

What is a vector?   102

What is WNV, and has it been around for very long?   103

WNV infects birds, horses, and humans—does it also multiply in mosquitoes?   104

What exactly is yellow fever virus?   106

What do we know about the global movements of arboviruses?   109

Do mosquitoes and ticks really carry needles? 110

What are the pandemic risks when it comes to these vectored viruses? 111

7 Single-Host Human Pathogens 114

Is an infection that is already widespread in humans likely to cause a pandemic? 114

What are noroviruses? 114

Are the noroviruses our only concern when it comes to the virus diarrheas? 115

What is intussusception? 116

Are there other ways of protecting against these viruses? 116

Apart from the hemorrhagic viruses, are cholera and typhoid the main causes of skin spots? 117

Is measles something that we should still be worried about? 118

Are there any other kinds of GI tract infections? 119

Is there a good hepatitis vaccine? 119

Are HepB and HepC the most dangerous of the hepatitis viruses? 121

Why is chronic hepatitis so dangerous? 122

Is it safe to have a blood transfusion? 123

Are any of these single-host human pathogens likely to cause pandemics? 124

8 HIV/AIDS 126

Is HIV still a concern? 126

Can what's happening now with HIV/AIDS be described as a pandemic? 127

Is there any improvement in the AIDS situation? 127

Where did this virus come from, and why didn't we see AIDS before 1981? 129

Was AIDS active much earlier in Africa? 130

Does the immune system fail totally when confronted with HIV? 131

How does HIV target the CD4+ T cell? 133

Do we yet have a vaccine for AIDS?   133

Will we ever have a vaccine for AIDS?   134

Has science failed us when it comes to HIV/AIDS?   135

What progress has been made in the last 25 years?   136

Could AIDS blow up in some way to cause an even bigger problem?   138

Once in the human body, can HIV ever be eliminated?   139

The Bottom Line   142

9 Mad Cows and Creutzfeldt-Jakob Disease   143

Has there ever been a mad cow or Creutzfeldt-Jakob disease pandemic? 143

So what is spongiform encephalopathy?   144

If the TSEs are infections, what's the big mystery?   145

Did BSE originate from sheep scrapie?   147

What is "bone meal"?   148

Has anyone contracted vCJD from eating imported British beef?   148

Was there even the possibility of a BSE/vCJD pandemic?   149

Does the history of BSE/CJD raise other concerns?   149

Are the TSEs a pandemic risk?   150

10 Economics and the Human-Animal Equation   152

What type of pandemic infection causes the most economic damage?   152

Is a novel respiratory infection the only economic threat?   153

Will it be massively expensive if quarantine officials are suddenly
faced with an emergency?   154

From a financial standpoint, does influenza remain our main concern?   155

Why is FMD so damaging?   156

Could there ever be a global FMD pandemic?   157

Has an animal virus ever been introduced deliberately into "virgin soil"? 158

Other than as a consequence of bioterrorism, is a veterinary
pandemic likely?   162

Are animal and human pandemics dealt with very differently?   165

Can returning tourists be infected with something that transmits
to animals?   166

Can imported animals infect humans?   166

Can humans be infected from imported animal or other products?   167

In Summary   168

11 Bioterrorism   169

Could sophisticated terrorists initiate a pandemic?   169

What about Saddam Hussein and his weapons of mass destruction?   171

Why is a rogue state more worrisome than a terrorist cell when
it comes to biological weapons?   171

Why would smallpox potentially be used in bioterrorism?   173

What do we know about anthrax?   175

Can you envision other novel bioterror pandemic scenarios?   177

Is a bioterrorist-initiated pandemic unlikely?   178

12 Protecting Humanity from and during Pandemics 179

Is there anything that I can do personally to limit the possibility of a
dangerous pandemic?   179

What if I become ill while traveling?   182

What if I develop symptoms after I return home?   182

Apart from being a responsible traveler, what else might I do?   184

Are there useful steps that I can take at the level of my local community? 186

How do I protect my family if a pandemic hits?   187

Does the idea of being "too clean" apply to pandemics?   190

Where do I look for help if I become infected during the course of a
major pandemic?   192

The Bottom Line   193

13 Conclusions   195

FURTHER READING   201

INDEX   213

ACKNOWLEDGMENTS

Though I've spent my whole research career working in the area of infection and immunity and have attended many broad-ranging scientific conferences and served on committees and task forces focused on issues to do with global infectious disease, my specific expertise is neither in public health nor in clinical medicine, both of which are obviously central to this book. I am thus enormously grateful to colleagues who have given their time to critique some or all of these chapters. In this context, I give particular thanks to my infectious disease physician friends, Miguela Caniza, Graham Brown, Ian Gust, and Stephen Kent. Rob Webster and Anne Kelso scrutinized what I wrote about influenza and pandemics in general, while Colin Masters read the chapter on vCJD and mad cow disease. John Mathews provided useful comments on the overall theme. Illustrations have been sourced online from the CDC and the Images Archive at the National Library of Medicine, the WHO Regional Map is reproduced with permission from the WHO, and I thank my close colleague Rob Webster for the other material presented in the figures. I also thank my wife Penny for reading the text, editors Tim Bent and Keely Latcham at Oxford University Press, and my agent Mary Cunnane.

ABBREVIATIONS

AFRIMS   Armed Forces Research Institute for Medical Sciences

AIDS   Acquired immune deficiency syndrome, caused by HIV

B cells   Ig+ lymphocytes that become the antibody producing plasma cells

BCG   Bacillus Calmette Guerin, a TB vaccine strain

BSE   Bovine spongiform encephalopathy; mad cow disease

CCR5   Chemokine receptor 5, one of the two HIV receptor proteins

CCU   The British MRC Common Cold Unit on Salisbury Plain (now closed)

CD4   Surface protein marking "helper" T cells that promote immune responses

CD8   Surface protein on "killer" T cells that destroy virus-infected cells

CDC   The USPHS Centers for Disease Control and Prevention, Atlanta, GA

cDNA   Complementary DNA made from RNA using RT, for the PCR

CJD, vCJD   (variant) Creutzfeldt Jakob disease, a TSE

CMV	cytomegalovirus, or HHV5, a persistent herpesvirus
CO_2	Carbon dioxide
CoV	Coronavirus
COPD	Chronic obstructive pulmonary disease
CTL	Cytotoxic T lymphocyte, the same as a CD8+ killer T cell
DNA	Deoxynucleic acid; the hereditary material of some viruses and all cells
DHF	Dengue hemorrhagic fever
DOT	Direct observed treatment, for those with TB who may be non-compliant
EBV	Epstein Barr virus; causes infectious mononucleosis and some cancers
ECDC	European Centre for Disease Control and Prevention
ECMO	Extracorporeal membrane oxygenation, as in a heart/lung machine
ELISA	Enzyme-linked immunosorbent assay; detects antibodies by color change
FDA	U.S. Food and Drug Administration, which licenses drugs and vaccines
flu ABC	Influenza A, B, and C viruses
FMD	Foot and mouth disease, of cattle
GAVI	The private Global Alliance for Vaccines and Immunization
GI	Gastrointestinal; of the gut
GRID	Gay-related immunodeficiency disease, an early name for AIDS
H	Hemagglutinin protein, the primary target of flu-specific antibodies
HAART	Highly active antiretroviral therapy; multi-drug treatment to control HIV
HepA-E	Different viruses that cause human hepatitis
HHV	Human herpesvirus
HHV6&7	HHVs that cause human roseola infantum

Hi-path	High pathogenicity, or virulent, influenza A virus
HPAI	Hi-path avian influenza A virus
HIV	Human immunodeficiency virus, the cause of AIDS
HSV1&2	Herpes simplex virus variants causing cold sores (1) and genital issues (2)
IFN-	Interferon, a secreted defense molecule involved in virus control
Ig	Immunoglobulin, or antibody that may be of the IgG, IgE, or IgA class
KSHV	Cancer causing (in AIDS) Kaposi's sarcoma herpesvirus (HHV8)
LCMV	Lymphocytic choriomeningitis virus; a mouse virus that infects humans
Lo-path	Low pathogenicity, or mild, influenza A virus
LPAI	Lo-path avian influenza A virus
M2	The matrix 2 ion channel protein that is at low levels on flu viruses
mAb	Monoclonal antibody: Ig of a single specificity, made in hybridoma cells
MDR	Multi-drug-resistant TB, and other bacteria
MHV	Mouse hepatitis virus, a coronavirus
MRC	The British Medical Research Council, equivalent to the U.S. NIH
mRNA	Messenger RNA, the template for making proteins
MSM	Men who have sex with men
N	Neuramininidase, the second (with H) protein on flu viruses
NA	Nucleic acids, the hereditary template of life
NIAID	National Institute of Allergy and Infectious Disease, part of the NIH
NIH	National Institutes of Health, the U.S. funding agency for medical research
NPC	Nasopharyngeal carcinoma caused by EBV, mainly in ethnic Chinese
O_2	Oxygen

OIE	Organization Internationale des Epizootiques, UN agency in Paris
OPV	Oral polio (Sabin) vaccine
PCR	Polymerase chain reaction for expanding viral, and other, NA sequences
PEPFAR	President's Emergency Plan for Aids Relief; supplies drugs to the poor.
PM	Post mortem
Polio	Poliomyelitis, or infantile paralysis, caused by a picornavirus
PrP	Prion protein, the cause of the TSEs including BSE, CJD, and vCJD
PUO	Pyrexia (fever) of unknown origin
RBC	Red blood cell, or erythrocyte that carries O_2 around the body
RHD	Rabbit hemorrhagic disease, caused by a calicivirus
RNA	Ribonucleic acid, the hereditary material on many of the smaller viruses
RRV	Ross River virus, an Australian alphavirus
RT	Reverse transcriptase, a virus enzyme copies RNA back into DNA
SARS	Severe acute respiratory syndrome, caused by a bat CoV
SCC	Squamous cell carcinoma, in the liver of HepB and HepC cases
SiRNA	Small interfering RNA, a molecular regulator
SIV	Simian immunodeficiency virus, causes AIDS in some monkeys
SSPE	Subacute sclerosing panencephalitis, caused by defective measles virus
SW	2009 H1N1 swine flu pandemic virus
T1/2	Half-life, typically of a drug or injected monoclonal antibody in blood
TB	Tuberculosis; lung disease caused by *Mycobacterium tuberculosis*

T cells	Thymus-derived lymphocytes, sets of circulating white blood cells
TDR	Total drug resistant, particularly TB
TSE	Transmissible spongiform encephalopathy, caused by PrPs
TTSH	Tang Tock Seng Public Hospital, Singapore
UN	United Nations
USAMRID	U.S. Army Medical Research Institute for Infectious Disease
USPHS	United States Public Health Service
WBC	White blood cell: moncocytes, neutrophils, T&B lymphocytes, and more
WHO	World Health Organization of the UN
WNV	West Nile virus
XDR	Extreme drug resistant TB, and other bacteria
YFV	Yellow fever virus

INTRODUCTION

Pandemic—we react immediately and viscerally to the word, which seems so close to "panic," though they actually share no etymological connection ("panic" derives from the Greek mythological creature Pan). But pandemics can cause panics, and the sense of imminent danger may be more universally contagious than any virus or bacterium. A lethal virus spreading rapidly and inexorably is, to most of us, a truly terrifying thought, so much so that it pushes other nightmare scenarios that generally hover at the edges of our consciousness (terminal cancer, leukemia, incipient dementia, stroke, quadriplegia, cardiomyopathy, and so on) into deep background. Still, should a pandemic hit, it's essential that we don't go into panic mode. We need to keep our wits about us.

This book is intended to help in that cause. Rather than focusing on the high drama that goes with chasing down dangerous pathogens, the basic intent is to supply accessible information about what's out there and what we should do when a threat emerges. While my personal involvement with infectious diseases is laboratory based, I've had a lot of help from medical friends who deal with the clinical and public health realities. Then, as a research investigator and nonfiction science writer who has increasingly been drawn into various public debates, I'm also very conscious that an acute sense of dread can seize some of my fellow citizens, including many who are well educated, when it comes to understanding the intricacies of disease processes. Some experience a gut-wrenching sense of revulsion when they encounter technical terms. This book contains a few. But I hope that readers won't simply give up when they come across the first bit of scientific jargon. To understand both infections and what to do about them, we need to know something of the vocabulary that's used by the professionals. I do my very best to explain matters in an accessible way, beginning with a synopsis of infection and immunity, the basis of any discussion of pandemics. And in the hope that you will be persuaded to persist with that little science/technology tutorial, I've also included a few human stories and even the occasional outrageous statement.

We all benefit from understanding at least a little about the various viruses, bacteria, and other bugs that have the capacity to live in and on us. After all, they are in many senses our most intimate associates. When a head cold or mild flu-like illness spreads, we experience a gentler form of what would happen when a genuine pandemic virus comes on the scene. It is my hope that what you encounter in the pages that follow will provide useful background, such that you have enough information to refine your search when you look up your symptoms on the Web, or hold your own when you get involved in a discussion of vaccination, or know what to expect when you travel to regions where dangerous pathogens are circulating. Readers with some background in biology or medicine may feel tempted to skip this brief summary, though I must confess that as I went about the process of checking some of my facts, I realized that there were some points on which my understanding was flawed, and I've been doing research on infection and immunity for 50 years.

A word about medical terms that are in common use but not always understood. I will, for instance, be talking about two "syndromes," as in SARS (severe acute respiratory syndrome) and AIDS (acquired immunodeficiency syndrome). A syndrome is a complex, newly recognized condition about which we know the "what" but not the "why," though the label often sticks after we do work out the "why." A familiar example is Down syndrome, a developmental abnormality associated with the presence of all, or part of, an additional 21st chromosome. First described in 1866 by the British physician John Langdon Down, it took almost a century to establish the genetic basis of this characteristic condition. Though such names are firmly embedded in clinical practice, modern, evidence-based medicine identifies new diseases by their known cause (etiology) rather than by the name of an eminent doctor or by some symptomatic shorthand. The cause of SARS, for instance, was soon worked out, though not before the disease had achieved broad notoriety. Given the incredible speed of contemporary communication and the short media cycle, the "syndrome" label was firmly fixed in both the public consciousness and the scientific literature.

"Syndrome" therefore reflects that first phase of confusion and, to some degree, fear. When the SARS outbreak seemed to strike out of nowhere in the early years of the twenty-first century, the citizens of Hong Kong and Singapore were terrified. The infection spread extremely fast. People stopped traveling. The effects on local businesses were disastrous (except those selling disinfectants and protective facemasks). The hotels reported immense financial losses. That was also true for airlines. While SARS was essentially dealt with—identified and contained—in the course of six to eight months, the economic consequences were still being felt two years later.

Rational thinking can quickly be compromised by pervasive fear, even when the situation may not be all that bad. I happened to be in Toronto in October 2009 when an otherwise healthy and active teenage boy died of the pandemic H1N1 influenza A virus, known now as the "swine flu." People were deeply shocked and, as the vaccine against this virus was just becoming available, rushed to have their kids immunized. But the logistics of vaccine delivery and the amounts at hand meant that not every child could be protected immediately, a fact that caused general outrage, with parents demanding that the government increase the supply without delay. Yet, six months later, when most had concluded that the "swine flu" caused a generally mild infection, it was hard to give the vaccine away, even to pregnant women who were, and remain, at significant risk.

As an active member of two research programs (one in Memphis, Tennessee, the other in Melbourne, Australia) that focus on influenza immunity, I was very aware of the efforts being made to sort out the identity of this novel—meaning, as it sounds, previously unknown—version of a familiar pathogen. Both teams contributed significantly to the understanding that some components of the H1N1 "swine flu" virus had been hiding out for more than 90 years in our fellow mammals. The strain that emerged so suddenly in early 2009 was born when two different viruses that infect pigs got mixed up together—a process called "reassortment"—to produce a pathogen that spread rapidly in humans. Looking at the gene sequences of the new virus, scientists soon realized that at least one of the major proteins is very similar to that found by Jeffrey Taubenberger and his colleagues in the "resurrected" genome (completed in 2005) of the virus that caused the 1918 Spanish flu pandemic. While we can't yet reproduce the scenario in Michael Crichton's *Jurassic Park* and bring complex creatures like dinosaurs back from the dead, Taubenberger and colleagues were able to recover virus gene sequences from several different sources of human post-mortem material. These were then "stitched together" to remake the pathogen that caused the Spanish flu, which remains the worst pandemic of modern times. That 1918 "Lazarus" virus is handled under ultra-high-security conditions, for although we know a great deal about these pathogens, there remains much that is not understood about why people die from influenza.

Most of us now associate "pandemics" with "influenza," reflecting the fact that all four acutely lethal pandemics experienced (thus far) in the twentieth and twenty-first centuries (see Figure I.1) have involved the flu. While the very first flu virus was not isolated until 1933, influenza (sometimes known by its French term, *la grippe*) has long been familiar and is

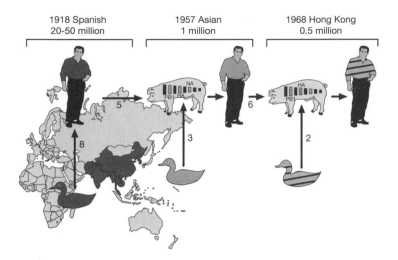

Figure I.1. This summarizes the three influenza A virus pandemics of the twentieth century and illustrates their possible origins, either directly from an avian species (1918), or as a consequence of viruses that are circulating in birds, humans, and/or pigs coming together in the lung of a pig. The small rectangles in the pig symbolize the 8 influenza gene segments that can reassort (mix and match) if a pig lung cell is infected simultaneously with two different viruses to give a novel pathogen that is highly infectious for us, a process called "antigenic shift." The broad virus types are categorized by the numbers assigned to the surface hemagglutinin (H) and neuraminidase (N) proteins present on the outside of the virus particles. The common names given to these viruses reflect where the pandemic was first acknowledged (in 1918) or the virus was initially isolated (1957 and 1968), and the counts below are for those who are thought to have died in the first year or two of virus circulation. Seasonal variants that arise from mutational change ("antigenic drift") in the surface H3 and/or N2 proteins of the Hong Kong flu virus are still circulating in us, with one such strain being the primary cause of the epidemic declared for the United States in January 2013.

Reproduced courtesy of Dr. Robert G. Webster at St. Jude Children's Research Hospital.

clearly described in records dating from the Renaissance and even before. Following the discoveries of Louis Pasteur, Robert Koch, and other nineteenth-century microbiologists, the basic nature of infectious disease was widely understood by the time that European nations and their colonial cousins embarked on that appalling tragedy of 1914–1918, the Great War. According to an account written later by Quartermaster General Erich von Ludendorff, the joint German military commander (with

Field Marshall Paul von Hindenburg), the Spanish flu pandemic helped bring the conflict to an end by further depleting the ranks of the armies. German manpower was rapidly exhausted, and America's entry into the war meant that Hindenburg and Ludendorff were facing what seemed like an endless reserve of fresh troops.

Though initially the Allied and Axis politicians and generals weren't admitting to the disease's effects, the Spanish, who were non-combatants, did the right thing—in the public health sense—and acknowledged that influenza was rampant. Spain gets a bum rap for being open about this. As John Barry describes in *The Great Influenza* (see "Further Reading" list), the virus likely came across to Europe with the newly arriving (from June 1917) American Expeditionary Force. While it was known by the 1930s that the Spanish flu was indeed caused by an influenza A virus, the specific characteristics of this deadly pathogen remained unclear until Taubenberger and his colleagues brought it "back to life" from lung tissue that had been stored for 80-plus years.

The shock of the worst pandemic of modern times was initially blunted by the sheer horror of what had happened in the trenches and battlefields of Belgium and France. In fact, many more were to succumb to influenza than were killed by bombs, bullets, poison gas, diarrhea, bacterial infections like gas gangrene, or simply drowning in the thick mud of Flanders. As described in a contemporary account by physician Victor Vaughan, the bodies of American recruits were "stacked about the morgue like cords of wood," and yet the full extent of the catastrophe was initially concealed for reasons of military security. But the story soon got out and, by the time the Spanish flu hit civilian populations, the fear was palpable. In the end, as many as 50 million people died.

Could the same thing happen today? Modern air travel means that the dissemination of the equivalent of the 1918 virus would be worldwide, perhaps within a matter of weeks. Given that the global population is about four times greater than it was back then, we could be looking at a mortality rate in excess of 100 to 200 million. That's one scenario. The other is that because of modern medicine the reemergence of a Spanish-like flu virus might not be so lethal. Many who have looked back at the detailed medical and pathology records from that time think that a significant proportion (if not the majority) of the deaths in 1918–1919 were due to the exacerbating effects of bacterial infections that became established on top of the initial, virus-induced lung damage. If such secondary bacterial pneumonia was, indeed, to be a major cause of severe disease in a contemporary influenza pandemic, substantial numbers could be saved by the judicious use of antibiotics, even if the virus spread widely before a vaccine became available.

Perhaps because of the profound trauma associated with the Great War—which obliterated an entire generation of French, German, and British young men (and killed 116, 516 Americans with more than 320,000 casualties)—there is little in the contemporary literature of the 1920s and 1930s that tells of the devastation caused by the flu pandemic. The medical and scientific accounts of the time are written in the dispassion-ate style of the physician, pathologist, or public health service doctor. As ever, to appreciate the human dimension, we look as much to creative writing as to analytical descriptions by sci-entists and popular syntheses by nonfiction authors. Katharine Anne Porter's 1939 novella *Pale Horse, Pale Rider* gives us an acute sense of the grief and loss borne by those who sur-vived. More recently, Dennis Lehane's *The Given Day* (2008) interweaves influenza, baseball, Babe Ruth, and the political machinations and corruption affecting the Boston municipal administration and police force. Lehane gives a sense of the courage of the public officials who, though poorly paid, put their lives at risk to help the sick, and describes how some who survived the infection were unable to work again and died young. Published in 2012, Tom Keneally's *The Daughters of Mars* puts a human face to the disastrous loss of nursing staff as influenza compromised all aspects of the war on Europe's

Western Front. Excellent factual treatments include Alfred Crosby's classic *America's Forgotten Pandemic: The Influenza of 1918* (first published in 1976) and the aforementioned *The Great Influenza* (2004) by John Barry, both of which convey the deep rips that the pandemic inflicted in the social fabric.

Photographs of the time, looked at closely, give a sense of scale. There are those showing seemingly endless rows of white-sheeted beds in massive infection wards. Others show streets packed with people wearing one of those minimally effective cloth surgical masks (Figure I.2). People were fined when they ripped them off and danced in the streets to celebrate Armistice Day, November 11, 1918. The authorities, realizing the scope of what they were facing, didn't ask recovered (or as yet unafflicted) municipalities to help by providing more doctors. In any case, largely as a consequence of the demands

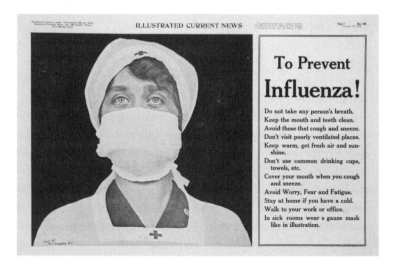

Figure I.2. The advice given in this 1918 poster from Connecticut is as apt today as it was then, with the possible exception that it may be better to take your own automobile than to walk. Back then, the authorities would have been thinking in terms of trains, buses and electric trolleys. Also, though fresh air and sunshine may make us feel good, it is unwise to access those in a crowded place if there is a raging flu or any other pandemic.

From the Image Archive at the U.S. National Library of Medicine.

of the war, physicians were in short supply and, during those very early days of the scientific medicine revolution (see Barry's book) that has led to such improved health outcomes in our time, there was not much that they could do for patients. Whether those with severe flu symptoms lived or died was largely independent of treatment.

What made the Spanish flu pandemic so terrible was that healthy people in the 20-to 40-year age groups were at high risk and, once infected, died with alarming speed. There are accounts of individuals first feeling ill at work, taking a trolley to go home, and being found dead at the end of the ride. Some went to bed feeling a bit "under the weather" and simply never woke up. Comparable symptoms have been seen in the relatively few human cases of H5N1 bird flu, which is still active in regions of Asia and remains a potential pandemic threat—perhaps the greatest of them all. This type of death is not characteristic of secondary bacterial disease, and it would not be prevented by antibiotic treatment.

In 1918, scientists did succeed in making a vaccine but, as they had not identified the cause of the infection, it proved useless. Together with reasonably good vaccines, there are now specific antiviral drugs for influenza, though they have to be taken very early in the course of the disease if they are to be of any value. Moreover, "escape mutants"—forms of the virus that are selected by the treatment—can quickly emerge for at least the H1N1 (Figure I.1) flu strains, the virus type that caused the Spanish flu. Indeed, apart from influenza, HIV, hepatitis C virus (very recently), and some of the herpes viruses, an unlikely cause of pandemics, there are no specific (as distinct from "symptomatic") therapies for virus diseases. That is certainly the case for the SARS, Hendra, and Nipah viruses, for example—all virulent pathogens that have recently "crossed" from some wild animal reservoir into the human population, though only the SARS virus adapted to cause substantial human-to-human spread. I will discuss all these infections in the chapters that follow.

Viruses, especially respiratory viruses, remain the greatest pandemic threat. We don't have to worry about—let alone
panic over—every pathogen that happens to be out there
somewhere, lurking, perhaps in a wildlife reservoir, perhaps in
some laboratory freezer. The websites of government agencies,
like the National Institute for Allergy and Infectious Diseases
(NIAID) and the Centers for Disease Control and Prevention
(CDC), which are charged with protecting the health of people
around the world, provide long lists of "Emerging Pathogens"
and potential "Bioterror Agents" that could cause terrible
diseases. You can look them up for yourself, if you're interested. Most of these "bad bugs" are, for one reason or another,
unlikely to break out and cause a pandemic. In fact, part of the
motivation behind this book is to allay concerns about widely
publicized infections, such as Ebola, Marburg, Sin Nombre,
West Nile, Nipah, Hendra, and so on—infections that might
cause horrific symptoms and suffering but are nonetheless
not obvious pandemic threats. Unless these pathogens change
(mutate) in some way that allows them to spread effectively
by aerosol/droplet exposure, we can limit the possible risk by
applying rigorous environmental control, sanitation, and isolation procedures.

Nearly a century after the Spanish influenza pandemic,
how prepared are we to handle an unpredicted challenge
from a virulent pathogen? The science of 2013 is vastly more
sophisticated than that of 1918—or, for that matter, of the
1980s, when we first became aware of HIV/AIDS, or even of
2002, when the hitherto unknown SARS virus emerged suddenly from its animal reservoir. However, what goes on in
the laboratory does not offer the whole story when it comes
to pandemics. The effectiveness of any response will depend
on the character and circumstances of those threatened.
Communities living in poverty are infinitely more vulnerable than the fortunate global minority (including those most
likely to read this book) who have ready access to extensive
medical and public health infrastructure. The best-protected

will be citizens of nation-states in which a strong sense of common purpose and shared responsibility prevail.

Nonetheless, even well-resourced and optimally organized societies would easily be overwhelmed by a real pandemic. A so-called "normal" influenza season, for example, may require the extensive use of critical care beds and "substitute lung" technology—breathing machines, effectively—to support those with severe pneumonia. Such resources are quickly stretched to the limit. In the face of a pandemic, patient triage would be inevitable, together with enforced limitations of personal movement and the organization of minimal human contact mechanisms for the distribution of food and other key supplies. As with major floods, earthquakes, and other forces majeures, the police, various emergency services, and the military (both full-time personnel and reservists) would soon be involved, providing specialists and equipment. Activating the military may sound alarmist, but fighting a pandemic is a form of war, with front lines, theaters of combat, and foot soldiers. Following the insights of von Clausewitz, those in command must be prepared both psychologically and practically to deal with a full spectrum of physical and sociopolitical realities.

As a species, we humans are programmed by our evolutionary history to respond rapidly to imminent threats, and we are capable of showing great altruism and courage. This was true during the Spanish flu pandemic and would be no less the case today. The city of Philadelphia, for example, was hit early and hard in 1918, with the consequence that the trained nurses available were soon worked to exhaustion. Student nurses were given the option to return home, but not one did. The 1919 School of Nursing yearbook for Philadelphia's University of Pennsylvania records the names of classmates Grace Fitzgerald and Marie Luise Boremann, who gave their lives on October 12 and 13, 1918. This tragedy was repeated again and again. For their service in naval hospitals in Philadelphia and Virginia, Marie Louise Hiddel, Edna Place, and Lillian Murphy were awarded the U.S. Navy Cross, posthumously.

Every crisis brings out the best and the worst of humanity—from heroism to opportunism. Both are illustrated in movies such as *Outbreak* (1995) and *Contagion* (2011). *Outbreak* may be good entertainment for horror-movie fans, but scientific integrity is sacrificed for dramatic effect. Steven Soderbergh's direction of *Contagion*, on the other hand, relied heavily on the advice of Columbia University infectious disease specialist Ian Lipkin and provides a generally believable overview of a worst-case pandemic. As the drama unfolds, the movie highlights the roles of public health officers, research scientists, informed citizens, the police, and the military in providing immediate protection and developing long-term solutions. What both films illustrate is that pandemics are inherently unpredictable. Neither human society nor the human immune system can be adequately prepared for them. Working in our favor, however, is more than a century of history and experience, together with the steady advance of science. Ironically, the latter may make us more preoccupied with pandemics than we actually need to be. Increasingly sophisticated diagnostic tools can lead to the declaration of a pandemic for an infection that spreads rapidly but poses no major threat. And if the whole thing turns out to be a squib—a false alarm—the inevitable media hype can create cynicism. Were those sounding the warning bells simply seeking to manipulate us and, perhaps, enhance their own importance and access to government resources? Such attitudes can be dangerous if they lead to outright indifference.

That would change quickly if people started to die. The sense of acute danger would return immediately. No book can, or should, fully assuage our fear of pandemics, but it can help us to respond appropriately. During the early phase of the 2009 flu pandemic, the "worried well"—as uninfected but anxious people are sometimes called—flooded the emergency outpatient clinic at the hospital down the street from my home in Melbourne. They no doubt thought this was a sensible thing to do. Actually, it wasn't. The mere act of coming together at a site where some are likely to be infected with a highly contagious virus would only serve to hasten its spread. While, of course, we need to remain engaged and informed, those of us who live in societies with a functioning health care system should not become too obsessed by the possibility of a global infectious disease crisis. Apart from cultivating sensible practices, such as vaccinating our children against the common infections of childhood and inculcating family routines that emphasize hand (and other) hygiene, the best we can do is to support the tax-base that funds the public health services, basic biomedical and epidemiological research, health care infrastructure, the police, and so forth.

In the developing world, on the other hand, pandemic infections can be superimposed on a background of malnutrition and other persistent problems, including HIV/AIDS, malaria, and roundworm infestations in children. The global poliomyelitis eradication initiative taught us that it is important to foster a capacity for vaccine production in countries where the disease is active, or to ensure that vaccines made elsewhere are culturally acceptable. The polio campaign was derailed in 2003, when a rumor spread in northern Nigeria that the standard, live polio vaccine that has been in use globally for decades had been engineered by the CIA to cause infertility in girls. As a consequence, people stopped vaccinating their children and the number of clinical cases tripled from about 350 in 2003 to 1140 in 2004. Furthermore, the disease spread beyond Nigeria and there were recurrences in 12 other African countries. That possibility of incursion from elsewhere is a major reason why kids in the advanced societies are still given the polio vaccine.

The situation was reversed for a time by manufacturing the vaccine in an Islamic country (Indonesia), an initiative that also fostered the development of a local vaccine industry. By 2010, there were only 48 Nigerian cases. Then the whole thing fell apart again from December 2102, when 16 dedicated (mainly young and female) workers involved in the poliomyelitis eradication campaign were murdered in Pakistan. Northern Nigeria soon followed suit, with the killing of 12 more vaccinators and three North Korean doctors. Somehow, if we are to eradicate poliomyelitis, we have to rebuild trust and assure people in cultures that are very different from our own that childhood vaccination is not serving the interests of some Imperialist Plot. But then we can't even convince many young, often well-educated (in the liberal arts sense) Western parents to vaccinate their children.

Clear, honest communication that does not discriminate or assign blame to those who might be at particular risk is critical whenever there is a substantial infectious disease threat. Things are much better in this regard than they were in the early days of the HIV/AIDS pandemic, when some disastrous mistakes were made about what should be done. The cause of the disease was not known, and the fact that it was associated with the gay community led to reactions from various interests groups—including the gays themselves who were understandably defensive—that were, at times, simply unhelpful and delayed appropriate action. If you doubt that, read Randy Shilts's 1987 nonfiction book, *And the Band Played on: Politics, People, and the AIDS Pandemic*, or watch the 1993 TV docudrama of the same name. Now, the ubiquitous cell phone is an enormously powerful weapon for getting good information out there.

The "softer" social and behavioral sciences can be as important as "hard line" laboratory research when it comes to fighting pathogens, particularly when it is a matter of convincing those who have power and influence in societies where the overall level of public education is low. Harm-reduction strategies worked out by outfits like Australia's Burnet Institute involve local political and religious leaders, police chiefs, traditional medical practitioners/witch doctors, and the realities of family/tribal structures. Culturally sensitive approaches are likely to work much better than rigid, "one-size-fits-all" directives.

My country of origin, Australia, will come up fairly often through these pages. This is not a reflection of national chauvinism on my part. Surrounded by oceans and the only single nation that occupies a continent—approximately the same size as the "lower 48" of the continental United States—Australia illustrates both the efficacy and limitations of stringent quarantine procedures practiced over the nearly two and a half centuries since European settlement. Australia also provides two unique case studies for what happens when lethal viruses are deliberately introduced into a totally unprotected population (wild rabbits, as it turns out, not people). In addition, being isolated at the "other end" of the world and with a pragmatic system of parliamentary governance and the rule of law, Australian public policy is often formulated with a good understanding of what has, or has not, worked well elsewhere. That isolation has, of course, been greatly diminished by rapid international air travel. The Spanish flu virus did not make landfall in Australia until 1919, while the 2009 H1N1 "swine flu," on the other hand, is now believed to have reached Melbourne before it was first detected in California and Mexico.

In the end, the best policy against pandemics rests in providing honest and open information, in efforts to improve the lives of every human being, wherever they live, and in pressing on with the basic and applied science of infection and immunity. "Forward defense" strategies practiced in the poorer countries of Sub-Saharan Africa by organizations such as the CDC, the European Centre for Disease Prevention and Control (ECDC), and the World Health Organization (WHO) of the United Nations protect all of us. Pandemics remind us in a very simple, direct, and brutal way that we share the same planet.

The world of infection is inexorably dynamic. As I finish this in March 2013, both North America and Europe have been experiencing substantial epidemics caused predominantly by variants of familiar, but different influenza viruses. Over the past few months, many across the world have been off sick for a few days because of a norovirus (a group of viruses that cause the food poisoning–like symptoms we call stomach flu) pandemic. Even when they "go global," such non-lethal, but nonetheless very discomfiting (vomiting) conditions seem to slip by the media because they rarely kill anyone and soon pass. Beyond that, when it comes to pandemics, the pathogen—the infectious cause—is only half the equation: the other half involves who we are and what we do.

Thinking that way should also cause us to extend our concern about pandemics to a much greater challenge—that of achieving a more equitable and environmentally sustainable earth. In the long term, it is on this achievement that our survival as a species will depend. Pandemics are only part of the story, and perhaps not even the scariest part.

The focus of this book is to review what has happened before, to discuss the strengths and limitations of systems currently in place, and to summarize how we might protect ourselves in the future. As you read on, the first chapter defines some key terms and gives basic insights into the nature of infectious organisms like viruses and bacteria, the ways that these bugs enter our body to cause disease, the immune responses that (hopefully) fight them off, and the vaccines, drugs, and other treatments that we use to protect us. We then consider what is meant by "pandemic," "epidemic," and "outbreak," and follow what happened when a completely novel pathogen jumped suddenly from wildlife into the human population in 2002. That SARS outbreak provided a timely warning of what can result from the fear of an unknown and rapidly spreading disease. Continuing with the theme of respiratory infections, I discuss tuberculosis (TB) and influenza, both of which constitute ongoing and familiar threats, with the latter, as I've said, representing the most likely cause of a future pandemic, though multi-drug-resistant TB hovers out there. The focus on animal reservoirs extends to a broader account of how infections can jump from small mammals to us. That in turn brings us to the subject of insect vectors and the infections they transmit from wildlife to humans, and between humans.

Two chapters are then devoted to reviewing the endemic status and the pandemic potential of viruses that are now maintained only in human populations, though these "single-host pathogens" may have crossed over earlier from other species. One is focused exclusively on the human immunodeficiency virus (HIV), which continues to devastate the poorer countries while infecting only a small minority in the wealthier nations. Next comes an "early warning" discussion of an odd class of transmissible agents—the prions that drove cattle mad and caused a fatal neurological disease in some who ate contaminated beef. The theme of economic loss mentioned briefly in regard to SARS is expanded for both medical and veterinary pathogens, together with a discussion of the importance of quarantine and the story of what happened when, in an effort to protect native flora and fauna and the agricultural industries, two extraordinarily lethal viruses were introduced deliberately into a "virgin soil" situation. Those wild rabbits mentioned earlier were the target population for these particular "bioterror" scenarios. Most humans are, of course, a lot smarter and better organized than the average bunny, but the way in which these infections spread reflects what occurred in medieval Europe and how diseases like measles and smallpox wiped out indigenous people after Columbus and those who followed came to the New World of the Americas. The final chapters consider the dangers posed by bioterrorists, and discuss how we might best protect ourselves, our families, and our communities when it comes to any pandemic situation.

The concluding text provides a summary of the main themes, plus a few brief statements concerning related issues. Finally, there is a "further reading" list. Where it seems appropriate, I also provide a short summary at the end of individual chapters. As part of the What Everyone Needs to Know series published by Oxford University Press, most of the book adheres to a "Question-and-Answer" format. Contained here are the questions I believe many might ask, and the best answers that I can provide.

Finally, as this book goes to press, the Chinese authorities are dealing with a completely new H7N9 influenza A virus that has so far killed 26 of the 126 people who are known to have been infected. Elderly males with other health problems have been particularly at risk. So far, there is minimal evidence of person-to-person spread, but the molecular sequence is such that it seems almost "poised" for transmission in humans. Evidence been found for the presence of this virus in pigeons and, though it is likely being spread from urban live-bird markets, the incidence of infection in domestic poultry species is surprisingly low. There has been a co-ordinated international response, and those responsible are currently preparing virus seed stocks for rapid vaccine production should that become necessary. There could not be a better illustration of how well we are now doing with virus diagnosis and preparedness, and how sudden the emergence of pandemic viruses can be.

PANDEMICS

WHAT EVERYONE NEEDS TO KNOW

1

INFECTION AND IMMUNITY

This chapter focuses on some key points and terminology that will hopefully give those who are unfamiliar with the science of infectious disease just enough information to understand what follows, or any public discussion of pandemics. But don't expect too much, either of yourself or of me. As you read on, it may suit you to skim over the top a bit when it comes to any more detailed discussion of underlying mechanisms, while at the same time taking on board any basic message that could help minimize future personal risk. We all do that: I doubt I'll ever grapple effectively with string theory! Also, as you read through this, you will run into terms—"antibody," for instance—that are described in more detail later. Just hold the thought, as we will never get anywhere if I keep covering the same ground.

Though starting with the basics, like what an "infection" is, might seem simplistic, if what can occasionally be encountered in the print and broadcast media is anything to go by, even the people to whom we look for reliable information can be extraordinarily uninformed when it comes to infection and immunity. Some TV newscasters and journalists, along with the researchers and the fact/language checkers who prepare or edit their copy, are apparently unaware of the difference between a virus and a bacterium. I've seen the malaria parasite referred to as a "virus," and a few commentators don't even seem to grasp the difference between a drug and a vaccine. That's a massive gap in understanding, as the underlying principles are fundamentally different. The language of science is usually (though not invariably) precise. If we don't state clearly what we are talking about, it's easy to get at cross-purposes. You may have some familiarity with much of what follows, but it could just be worth your while to scan through and ensure that we're on the same page.

What is the difference between a virus and a bacterium?

The most fundamental difference is that, while a single bacterium carries all the cellular machinery necessary for its own replication, the sub-cellular viruses depend on the energy and protein-processing mechanisms found, for example, in the various cells of our body. Many bacteria are also motile, that is, they have the capacity to move themselves around. Viruses, on the other hand, are essentially inert particles that simply go where the wind blows, so to speak, or where the slime (mucus, snot, phlegm) that has carried them out of the body is deposited, or floats as fine droplets, or aerosols. Many bacteria move via the action of tiny surface projections, called flagella, that sweep them along. Others, the spirochetes, are perfect spirals that can be seen to "corkscrew" when observed in a "wet" preparation through the high power of an optical microscope—fascinating to watch! Then, like snails, some secrete their own copious slime, which helps them to get around the neighborhood. Slime, or mucus, is a very important, and often somewhat neglected topic when it comes to infection.

Unlike the more active and independent bacteria, viruses (see Figures 1.1 and 1.2) are basically protected packages of genetic information (RNA or DNA) that must invade living cells in order to multiply. The RNA or DNA is protected by an outer layer (or layers); some viruses have an added external "envelope," which is principally protein (capsid) plus incorporated lipids (fats) and carbohydrates (sugars). Different viruses have evolved a variety

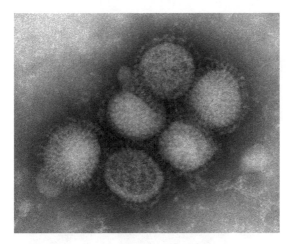

Figure 1.1. An electron micrograph of influenza A virus particles, with the surface H and N molecules fuzzily visible.

Public Health Image Library at the Centers for Disease Control

of mechanisms for entering a specific target cell, a process that is followed by un-coating to release their hereditary RNA or DNA into the cytoplasm. That instruction package (or genome) functions to redirect and exploit normal cellular processes, leading ultimately to the production of a new generation of virus particles (virions). The essential proteins and nucleic acids of these progeny virions are specified by the viral genome, while the lipids and carbohydrates are "borrowed" from the membranes of the host cell. With the influenza viruses, for example, that cycle from entry to maturity can take as little as 6 hours.

At the end of the replication cycle, there must be some mechanism to let the progeny virus escape so that more cells can be infected, either within the same or a different individual. Depending on the particular pathogen and cell type, virus release can involve the destruction (lytic death) of the original production factory, or the infected cell can coexist with the virus and continue to pump out new virions. This balance between lytic and persistent infection can be a major factor determining the severity, or virulence, of a particular pathogen. Soon, that

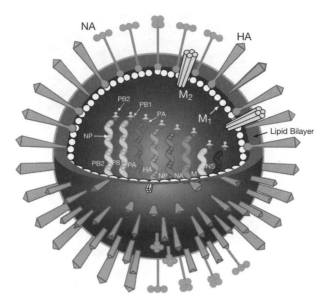

Figure 1.2. A diagram of the virus showing the 8 internal influenza virus genes and the HA (lozenge) and NA (stalk+3 dots) proteins protruding from the surface of the virus. The job of the HA (or H) molecule is to bind to any sialic acid (carbohydrate) on the outside of the cell so that the virus can attach and enter, while the NA (or N) neuraminidase enzyme breaks that bond for newly formed virus particles and allows them to escape so that they can infect other cells. New pandemic strains emerge when a different H type that is not recognized by preexisting serum antibodies circulating in large numbers of people comes in from another species. Also illustrated is the low abundance and highly conserved surface M2 ion channel protein, the target for some research groups that are trying to make cross-reactive influenza vaccines to provide protection against novel pandemic strains. Others are using genetic engineering approaches to modify, or shorten (truncate), the H protein so that the antibody response focuses on the conserved "stalk" region rather than, as is normally the case, on the more exposed, outer "head."

Courtesy Dr Robert G. Webster, St Jude Children's Research Hospital.

first invading virus has millions of progeny, each of which can infect and potentially destroy (or functionally compromise) another of our body's cells. That's why, as will be discussed later under immunity, it's so essential to knock out those virus factories as early as possible.

While every bacterium is clearly a living organism, there's an old debate (that's about as useful as the medieval theological discussion of "how many angels can fit on the head of a pin") asking whether we can truly describe viruses as being "alive." Come to your own conclusion: I don't find it particularly important. Just like all other life forms, bacteria have their own spectra of parasitizing viruses, called bacteriophages. The Latin *phage* means "eat," of course. Think *sarcophagus*, which means literally "flesh-eating stone." But just as a stone coffin doesn't really eat a human corpse—bacteria do that job—the bacteriophage kills (or persistently infects) rather than consumes its host.

As far as our health is concerned, bacteriophages may not be totally benign, as they can contribute to bacterial virulence. The childhood disease diphtheria is, in fact, caused by a strain of *Corynebacterium diphtheria* that carries a persistent bacteriophage with DNA encoding the diphtheria toxin. For more than 80 years, we have had a great vaccine that induces the production of antibodies for blocking (neutralizing) this toxin. With the collapse of the public health services that occurred soon after the demise of the Soviet Union, the number of deaths from diphtheria went up dramatically as children went unvaccinated. It is essential to immunize small children against diphtheria, whooping cough, and the other (formerly) common diseases of childhood.

And if you're wondering what the difference is between immunization and vaccination, there isn't one. I'll say more about immunity later in this chapter, but vaccination, from "vacca," the Latin for cow, is the older word, reflecting English physician Edward Jenner's 1796 scarification (scratching with a needle) of what is believed to be cowpox virus-infected material taken from a "blister" on the arm of a dairy maid, Sarah Nelmes, into the skin of eight-year-old James Phipps. Later challenged with the terrible (and closely related) human pathogen smallpox, or variola, James survived, as did Jenner's own son, who was also part of the experiment. Prior to Jenner's discovery, he and his contemporaries were following the practice of variolation, which probably originated in

China, whereby they did much the same thing with material from smallpox lesions (pustule, scab), relying on the fact that the route of inoculation and the age of the subjects (the young have better immune systems) allowed children to survive and to resist later exposure to the lethal, at worst, and disfiguring, at best (pockmarked faces), consequences of natural smallpox infection. That practice was brought to Boston in the seventeenth century by the Reverend Cotton Mather and was popularized by Dr. Zabdiel Boylston, with the consequence that many lives were saved during the course of an ongoing smallpox outbreak. Jenner's cowpox vaccination procedure was, of course, infinitely safer. Smallpox is the only human disease that we have ever eliminated (by vaccination) from the planet, with the WHO declaring in 1979 that the world is officially free of this terrible scourge. The vaccine that was used was not much more sophisticated than the original product available to Jenner!

Viruses and bacteria are everywhere. When we dive on a coral reef, for example, the seawater is loaded with bacteria and the phages that infect them but, fortunately, not us. Apart from the situation with C. diphtheria, the viruses that are of concern from the aspect of human health are the pathogens that invade and then multiply in anatomical sites like the surface epithelial cells of the mammalian respiratory tract (influenza, parainfluenza); the hepatocytes in our liver (yellow fever, hepatitis ABC); the white blood cells (HIV); and so on. Most bacteria, on the other hand, grow satisfactorily in cell-free, nutrient soups, from garbage-contaminated water to an open milk bottle left on a kitchen bench, to a "defined" culture medium in the laboratory. That's why you want to discourage any household practice of drinking directly from an open milk carton or juice container that is then returned to the refrigerator. No matter what toothpaste and/or mouthwash we use, our mouths are loaded with bacteria. In our body tissues, some pathogenic bacteria, like the TB organism, do enter (parasitize) our living cells, while others exist happily in our extracellular fluids.

Considering the broader environment, bacteria like the anthrax bacillus form resistant spores that survive indefinitely in soil, an option that is not available to viruses. When we step on a rusty nail, for example, the first question the doctor is likely to ask is: "How long has it been since you were vaccinated against tetanus?" If the answer is "way back," you will likely be given a booster dose of the vaccine (active immunization) or will be protected by the injection of immune serum. Such "passive" immunization is provided by antibodies circulating in the blood of humans or horses that have been vaccinated with the tetanus toxin. This need for immediate treatment reflects that a resistant form of the tetanus bacterium *C. tetani* is ubiquitous in the soil.

Everyone who watches the news on television has seen the three-second spot of a white-coated medical scientist feigning intense interest while holding a circular, flat plastic dish up to the light. The story line will likely be something to do with food poisoning (bacterial infection) from contaminated (usually fecal) vegetables, meat products or, perhaps, hen's eggs. In mid-2011, for example, *Escherichia coli* (*E. coli*)–contaminated bean sprouts from an organic farm in northern Germany caused 31 deaths and thousands of other infections. As with the 1918–1919 "Spanish" flu, Spain got the wrong end of the stick when Spanish cucumbers were wrongly blamed for the outbreak. Some organic farmers use a lot of cow manure, so it's advisable to wash such products well.

Returning to our plate-holding TV scientist, the lens of the videocam then focuses in on the exposed surface of the plastic plate to shows streaks (or lumps) of what is obviously bug growth on a translucent, or perhaps red or brown-colored, background. What you are seeing here is a Petri plate—named for German bacteriologist Julius Petri (1853–1921)—with bacterial colonies growing on nutrient, blood, or "chocolate" agar. Agar—the same stuff that's in ice cream—is made from seaweed, while the "nutrient" could be added protein, amino acids and vitamins (substrate looks translucent), fresh blood (red plate), or heated blood (chocolate plate). Much of the revolution in our understanding of infectious disease throughout the nineteenth century depended on the development of such bacterial culture media, either as fluid "soups" or in solid phase (Petri plates). If you think that sounds like cookery, you're right. The original insight for agar plates came from Fanny Hesse, who was working as a technician with her scientist husband in the laboratory of the great Prussian bacteriologist Robert Koch (1843–1910; Nobel Prize, 1905), who discovered *Bacillus anthracis* (anthrax), *Mycobacterium tuberculosis* (TB), and *Vibrio cholera* (cholera). Fanny Hesse was familiar with the use of agar in making jam!

This is a good point at which to relate just a little of the very early history of microbiology, the study of these very small bugs. Though we had known about unicellular life forms since the invention of the microscope by Antony van Leeuwenhoek (1632–1723), most believed that such life could be generated spontaneously from non-living material containing "pneuma," or "vital heat." That was disproved in 1859 by Louis Pasteur (1822–1895), who showed that a previously boiled "soup" in a standard flask left open at the top soon became turbid with contamination, while the same broth in an open, but "swan-necked" flask (where the dip in the neck meant that nothing could fall directly from the air into the fluid) remained clear. Pasteur, Robert Koch, and their colleagues then went on, through the course of the nineteenth century, to discover the basics of infection. A "must see" for any scientific tourist is the museum in Pasteur's own laboratory (including the original "swan neck" flasks) at the Institut Pasteur, Rue du Docteur Roux, in central Paris. Pasteur and his family lived in an apartment across the corridor from his lab, and he is entombed in the basement. Amazingly, in the 120,000 to 200,000-year-old history of humanity, we have understood infection for less than two centuries.

Also, it isn't just bacteria and viruses that we need to discuss when we're talking about subcellular (viruses) and unicellular (bacteria) infectious agents. I mentioned malaria a little earlier. Protists, more specifically protozoa like the malaria parasite, the trypanosomes—*Trypanosoma brucei* causes sleeping sickness—and *Entamoeba histolytica* (amebic dysentery) are also single cells. But, like us, protists/protozoa are eukaryotes, which means that they separate their DNA from the main substance of the cell (the cytoplasm) in a distinct, membrane-enclosed nucleus, while there is no such division in the prokaryote bacteria. There are many other differences, of course, including the fact that the protozoa often have very complex life cycles.

Algae—free-living protists that cause, for instance, toxic "blooms" in the oceans—and fungi, which range in size and complexity from the yeast-like *Pneumocystis carinii* that lives on the surface of our respiratory tract to mushrooms growing in a paddock, are also eukaryotes. As any Italian food fan knows, *con funghi* means "with mushrooms." Fungi, or molds, make many of the antibiotics (penicillin, streptomycin) that we, like them, use to kill off pathogenic bacteria. Some "industrial" microbiologists are focusing on the use of algae to "sequester" large amounts of carbon—taken in as the greenhouse gas CO_2—as a means of diminishing the extent of anthropogenic climate change. Others are trying to "scale up" algal systems for making carbon-neutral biofuels.

What is the difference between RNA and DNA?

We need to talk just a little about the genetic basis of life if we are to understand the difference between viruses versus bacteria, the protists and us. While the genetic information of bacteria and all higher life forms passes from generation to generation as DNA, viruses can have an RNA or DNA genome. What's the difference? Very briefly, the hereditary blueprint is written as a sequentially organized triplet code of nucleic acid base pairs, AU/CG (adenine-uracil, cytosine-guanine) for RNA and AT/CG (adenine-thymine, cytosine-guanine) for

DNA. When genes are read out in us, for example, the DNA code is "transcribed" to provide an RNA "message" (mRNA) that, in turn, serves as a template for assembling (translating) the appropriate sequence of amino acids, the building blocks of the proteins that are the basic structural and functional components of all life. It doesn't much matter for the purpose of the present discussion of pandemics if you don't understand the difference between RNA and DNA, apart from noting that some RNA viruses like flu and HIV throw off a lot of mutants as a consequence of lacking an adequate proofreading mechanism. Providing there is no "fitness" cost (failure to grow well), a single change in the AU/CG sequence can, for example, lead to escape from immune control. This happens much less readily for DNA viruses.

Over the past 30 years or so, advances like recombinant DNA technology have totally transformed both our understanding of, and the way we deal with, infections. This procedure involves the transfer of genetic material (including human DNA) into bacterial, yeast, insect, or, indeed, any cells that will grow as bulk cultures in stirred tanks or fermentation vats, and has greatly facilitated research on molecules that would, in days gone by, have only been available in very low concentrations. Being able to make such massive amounts of protein at will in bacterial systems has further enabled their direct use in, for example, a well-established vaccine that protects us against hepatitis B virus infection. In addition, after much effort by researchers, the popular media are now reporting that a new transduced-worm-cell strategy is working for influenza. I'm looking forward to seeing the data!

Our capacity to read out the nucleic acid sequences of RNA and DNA, or the amino acid sequences of proteins, has been enormously enhanced by developments in applied chemistry, robotics, computer technology, and engineering. While a decade back we would largely have relied on antibody tests (discussed later in this chapter) to look for, say, mutant viruses, the technology for "deep sequencing" is now so advanced that we analyze the virus nucleic acid code directly to see where any changes may have occurred. That's one reason that major state-of-the art reference laboratories play an ever increasing part in protecting us against diseases like influenza.

Many great advances in both diagnosis and research also depend on a spectacular transformative discovery: the poly-merase chain reaction, or PCR. This is the method that forensic scientists use to identify murderers and rapists from a spot of blood or semen and, conversely, has led to the release of wrong-fully convicted innocents who were serving life sentences or being held on death row pending execution for such crimes. You may have seen the 2010 Hollywood movie *Conviction*, in which the character played by Hilary Swank was able to use the results of PCR and gene sequencing from blood-contam-inated clothing to get her brother (played by Sam Rockwell) released for a murder committed before the PCR technique was invented.

The PCR principle was discovered in 1983 by Kary Mullis, the 1993 Nobel Prize winner for Chemistry, who tells the story in his entertaining autobiography *Dancing Naked in the Mind Field*. I won't go into the technical details but, by making "primers" that define either end of the genetic region of inter-est, the PCR approach allows the definitive characterization of the particular life form. If (as is the case for influenza) we are looking at an RNA virus, the genetic material is first cop-ied back to make a complementary cDNA using the enzyme reverse transcriptase (RT). The RT-PCR approach is also used to identify which genes are being "read-out" in a "normal" cell at any one time by expanding a cDNA copy of the mRNA template for making proteins. The discovery that RNA tumor viruses use RT to insert their genetic information into the ver-tebrate genome earned U.S. researchers Howard Temin and David Baltimore the 1975 Nobel Prize for Medicine. This led to the adoption of the term "retrovirus" and, when HIV emerged in the 1980s, allowed us to understand immediately how this virus, though it does not directly cause cancer, integrates into human DNA. Most viruses don't do this, and, when they are eliminated by the immune response, it is generally thought that none of their genetic information is retained in the recovered individual.

A thermal cycler, the relatively inexpensive piece of apparatus that allows the PCR to proceed, can be found in every "state of the art" biology laboratory throughout the world. The method uses a heat-resistant DNA polymerase, an enzyme (protein) that drives DNA replication to expand the nucleic acid sequences via successive cycles of heating and cooling. Then, if we know what we're looking for, the expanded product can be readily identified using a specific diagnostic kit involving, perhaps, something as simple as a change of color that can be assessed visually. On the other hand, if we were trying to identify a murder suspect or a novel variant of a pathogenic virus, it would be necessary to go to the more expensive alternative of gene sequencing to determine the exact nucleic acid sequence of one or more key gene segments.

Before PCR came on the scene, diagnostic microbiologists and virologists would have had to grow the organism in some sort of culture system (soups or plates for bacteria, living organisms such as baby mouse brain or cell cultures for viruses) and then use specific reagents, like antibodies to known viral proteins, to determine what it was that they had found. Antibodies are present in serum, and the term "serotypes" may still be used to describe variants of a particular pathogen. Now, PCR allows us to detect the tiniest amounts of viral genome and determine the exact identity within a matter of hours, or at most a day or two. The major influenza centers, for example, use expensive equipment that allows the immediate expansion, then sequencing, of large numbers of virus specimens. This means that we can track the progress of an influenza outbreak or pandemic with extraordinary precision, while at the same time monitoring for "escape mutants" that might be drug resistant, or show changes that could mean they will no longer be neutralized by circulating antibodies generated in response to the currently utilized vaccine.

Aren't viruses also much smaller than bacteria?

Yes, it's generally the case that viruses are smaller. As with bacteria, viruses carry the genes coding for particular structural proteins, such as the ribonucleoprotein that "wraps" and protects the influenza virus RNA and enzymes like reverse transcriptase and the polymerases necessary for reproduction (Figure 1.2). But viruses can be much more compact than bacteria. Their parasitic lifestyle means that they don't need to lug large organelles—the mitochondria that control energy metabolism and the ribosomes necessary for protein assembly—around with them. In fact, the first classification that divided bacteria and viruses back in the early decades of the twentieth century was based on findings that all the then known viruses (and no bacteria) passed through filters with a pore size around 220 nanometers (nm = 10^{-9} meters), or less. The smallest viruses get down to 17 nm, many are around 100 nm, and the biggest that commonly infect us (like the DNA cytomegalovirus) are 150–200 nm. For the early infectious disease researchers, "filterable" and "virus" went together like "gin and tonic." The word "virus" comes from the Latin *contagium vivum fluidum* (soluble living germ) coined by the eminent nineteenth-century Dutch microbiologist Martinius Beijerinck, who concluded that, after passing the infectious entity he was studying (now called tobacco mosaic virus) through a very fine filter, he was dealing with something liquid in nature.

To put the size of viruses in perspective, the diameter of the head of a pin is about 2 mm (or 2,000,000 nm), while the biggest spheroidal viruses that infect us are about 200 nm across. Calculating on the basis of surface area through the center, we could fit about 100 million virus particles on the head of a pin. That's a pretty rough calculation. Pinheads aren't likely to be completely flat, we haven't allowed "packing room," and only some viruses are regular in shape.

Electron microscopy has also established that the largest viruses are not so very different in size from the smallest bacteria. For example, the bacterium *Mycoplasma genitalium* can be just 200–300 nm, depending on its nutritional state. And, while most bacteria may be at least 1,000 nm, some of the filamentous filoviruses (like Ebola) can, though only 80 nm in diameter, be hundreds, or even thousands, of nm long. Recently, two newly discovered groups of viruses, the mimiviruses and megaviruses, have been found to be 400+ nm, raising speculation that they started out as bacteria, but have devolved to being parasites by kicking out the cellular machinery they find and exploit in some other cell type that now serves as their host.

Even so, it is the case that many of the bacteria that infect us are, after staining with mixes of vital dyes like May Grunwald/Giemsa (methylene blue/eosin/azure B, and named after the people who developed it), big enough to be seen via the high power of an optical microscope; this is not the case for the great majority of viruses. And, because bacteria could both be seen and grown in or on inert substrates while the still invisible viruses of vertebrates were known only to replicate in living animals, research on bacterial diseases moved much more quickly than the study of virus infections until the second half of the twentieth century.

The exception was the study of bacteriophages, as the bacterial targets were readily grown as "lawns" on inert, non-living substrates like nutrient agar plates, allowing the first serious analyses of virus mutants. Animal virology jumped forward in the 1930s with the adoption of embryonated hen's eggs as convenient "culture vessels" (see my book *Their Fate is Our Fate: How Birds Foretell Threats to Our Health and Our World*) to support the growth of many viruses that infect us. Most influenza vaccines are, for example, still made from virus produced in live chick embryos, though that era may be coming to an end. Then came the development of mammalian tissue culture (greatly aided by the availability of antibiotics to control bacterial contamination) in the 1950s, the necessary prerequisite for Jonas Salk (1955) and Albert Sabin (1957) to make the inactivated (Salk) and live/attenuated (Sabin) poliomyelitis vaccines that we still use today.

Why is it important to distinguish viruses from bacteria when discussing pandemics?

There are a number of reasons, such as the capacity of some bacteria to survive as resistant spores and so forth, but the really important difference rests in just one word: antibiotics. Looking back to the bad infections of the nineteenth century and earlier, it is obvious that a whole spectrum of bacterial diseases dominate the scene. Starting from the fourteenth century, the plague caused by the bacterium *Yersinia pestis* devastated Europe for centuries and regularly killed from one-third to one-half of those in a given town or village. Large numbers of men and women—including Winston Churchill's father, Lord Randolph—developed chronic neurological problems culminating in insanity as a consequence of being infected with the spirochete *Treponema pallidum*, the cause of syphilis. Bacterial diarrheas and fevers like cholera (*Vibrio cholerae*) and typhoid (*Salmonella typhi*) were a continuing scourge, while the devastation caused by tuberculosis (*Mycobacterium tuberculosis*) and leprosy (*M. leprae*) is vividly depicted in literature, from Biblical times to the late 1800s and beyond. Now, the sanatoria where TB patients were kept to experience the healing properties of fresh mountain and rural air have largely closed, along with the lazarets (human quarantine stations) and leper colonies. Though we worry about multi-drug-resistant TB and other bacteria, these have yet to cause epidemics in well-organized societies, though can be a major problem in hospitals and they do constitute a potential, global threat.

While the control of both bacterial and viral diseases benefited from improved public health measures (like cleaning up the water supply) and we saw the progressive development of effective vaccines to protect against at least some bacteria and viruses, there's a fundamental difference in the availability of therapeutic approaches (drugs) to cure those who do become infected. As we've discussed, bacteria, like protozoa and fungi, are cells in their own right that tend to cause disease relative to their numbers, location, and possible toxin production. The biochemical pathways common to many bacterial pathogens are sufficiently different from those used in our own cells to allow them to be blocked by the use of specific chemicals, first the sulfonamides (in the 1930s), then the antibiotics (from the 1940s). As a consequence, so long as the diagnosis is made before too much damage is done, medical professionals can usually counter any familiar or novel bacterial pathogen both rapidly and effectively with products that are currently available "off the shelf." Antibiotic resistance may ultimately develop, but by then both the condition and the cause will be more than familiar.

We can't yet use the same "blockbuster bomb" strategy to defeat viruses, as the drug in question could be as toxic for our own cells as it is for the pathogen. As a consequence, unlike the situation for bacteria and fungi, there are no "broad spectrum" treatments that function to defeat a whole range of different viruses. The net result is that antiviral drugs and specific "biologicals" (products made by living cells) like therapeutic monoclonal antibodies need to be targeted directly at gene products encoded by the individual pathogen. Small molecule antivirals (synthetic drugs made by chemists) have been developed with great success to control persistent infections like HIV and, more recently, hepatitis C virus and for the acute treatment of influenza (Figures 1.1 and 1.2), but the economic cost of producing such reagents for more severe, or less common infections is generally prohibitive. Hopefully, it will continue to be the case that there are few conditions like HIV/AIDS for which a cocktail of three drugs must be taken continuously for life. In the early days when the western pharmaceutical industry controlled the patents, these drugs were certainly great moneymakers for those companies.

Differential diagnosis is also a big problem for antiviral drugs, which we know, from the influenza experience, must be administered early if they are to be of any value for controlling a rapidly developing lytic infection. That will not, of course, be an issue if we are facing a pandemic with a known cause, a process of identification that, with modern technology, should take no more than a few days. But, in the absence of information that there is a particular pathogen on the loose, think about the situation facing a medical doctor in her consulting room as she tries to help some coughing, sneezing lump of human misery. There are literally hundreds of possibilities.

The key message here is that a whole lot of very different viruses can cause similar symptoms, reflecting that the ways that our infected cells and tissues respond are much less diverse than the array of potential pathogens. Unless there's an ongoing outbreak caused by a known virus, doctors can't tell the difference without some sort of specific, rapid test. Treating with a drug that stops the flu virus in its tracks will, for example, have no effect on a coronavirus or an adenovirus. One strategy that we might think about for blunting the impact of possible future pandemics is, though, to develop and test drugs targeting families of closely related viruses that could be potential threats. The neuraminidase inhibitors *Relenza* and *Tamiflu* can, for example, be used to limit infections with all influenza viruses, though there is the problem that drug-selected escape mutants may rapidly emerge.

Are colds and flu caused by hundreds of viruses?

Yes, if we're talking about coughs and sneezes and mild flu-like symptoms, not the "monster flu" that can kill us. We discuss that in more detail later. Improvements in tissue culture technology from the 1950s, then PCR, led to the identification of enormous numbers of candidates—rhinoviruses, enteroviruses, adenoviruses, paramyxoviruses, coronaviruses, metapneumoviruses, and so forth—that cause discomfiting but non-lethal infections confined generally to the upper respiratory tract (nose and pharynx).

And don't freak out, or look for any deep meaning, when you encounter different virus group names as you proceed through this text. While some have an obvious derivation— *rhino* is the ancient Greek for "nose," and the common cold rhinoviruses grow mainly in the nose—most are just classifications that link pathogens with similar molecular and (often, though not always) disease-causing profiles. There's not space in this book to go into the details, and it would be much, much more than you ever need to know. Think in terms of families like the Montagues and Capulets if you're a Shakespeare fan, the Ravenswoods and Lammermoors if Donizetti is your thing, or Ferraris and Maseratis if you're an up-market revhead. After all, most of us don't ask what a surname means when we meet someone for the first time, and even car enthusiasts may be content to just see the name badge of a classic automobile.

The story of how the common cold viruses were discovered and then researched is an interesting one. After the end of World War II, English virologist Sir Christopher Andrewes took over a U.S. "gift" facility, the prefabricated American Red Cross/Harvard Hospital, to found the British Medical Research Council (MRC) Common Cold Unit (CCU) on Salisbury Plain. Under Andrewes and the subsequent leadership of David Tyrrell, the CCU used human volunteers to establish that these generally mild but annoying respiratory infections are caused by many viruses, including the 100 or so human rhinoviruses that will only grow outside the body in tissue cultures maintained at the lower temperature of the nose. Though no vaccines were developed because of the great variety of possible causes, by the time the CCU closed in 1989, we had a much better understanding of the common cold. The paid volunteers came in groups of 30 or so at fortnightly intervals and, as the accommodation was warm and there were games to play and books to read, it was generally regarded as a good holiday by the impecunious students of that era. You can see some of these creatures from a very different world by looking at the short movie accessed via the website listed in the references. That also shows you how virologists worked way back then on open bench tops, with little of the protections mandated today. Among other things, the volunteers established that colds are not normally spread by kissing, or result primarily from sitting in a draft. If you think all science is super-sophisticated, a primary read-out for assessing the severity of these infections was to count the number of snotty, discarded paper tissues.

What exactly is a pathogen?

A true pathogen, whether it be a virus, a bacterium, or a protozoan, is a *virulent*, or *pathogenic*, infectious agent that causes obvious disease. The infection can be *systemic* (disseminated throughout the body via the blood circulation) or *localized* to a particular cell type or body organ. Some influenza viruses—which are prominent in any discussion of pandemics—cause mild, localized (to the gut in birds or to the lung in us) infections that are described as *lo-path* (low pathogenicity). Flu viruses that mutate to greater virulence and may, for example, spread to the brain are called *hi-path*. Specifically with respect to the H5N1 avian influenza (AI) viruses, you may encounter the terms HPAI (hi-path) and LPAI (lo-path) in media reports. Sometimes a given virus can be hi-path in one species (HPAI H5N1 flu in geese and swans) and lo-path in another (the same virus in ducks), which, as the birds are well enough to fly long distances, greatly increases the likelihood of national and international spread along normal migration pathways.

At any rate, the words "pathogenic" and "pathogenicity" derive from the scientific discipline of *pathology*: the study of the biological mechanisms fundamental to disease. In setting out to analyze how an infectious agent induces the tissue and organ pathology (abnormality and loss of function) that leads to severe symptoms, the research pathologist aims to tease out the *pathogenesis* of the underlying disease process. Typically, a medical pathologist who focuses on infectious pathogens will be the white-coated professional who gives the final word after a series of investigative steps that begin in the post mortem (PM) room and involve other highly trained professionals, like bacteriologists, virologists, or mycologists (who study fungi), all of whom are lumped under the general job description of microbiologist.

Just about everyone is familiar with forensic pathologists from reading the novels of Kathy Reich and Patricia Cornwell, or watching TV programs like *CSI* (CBS) or *Silent Witness* (BBC). While perhaps not as photogenic as TV actors, those who do PMs on, for instance, non-human primates infected with an extremely virulent virus like Ebola will be working under the high-drama conditions illustrated in movies like *Contagion*. All known infectious organisms are classified on a danger scale ranging from Biosafety Level (BSL) 1 to 4. Ebola virus is, for example, a BSL-4 organism that has to be handled in a BSL-4 facility. This means that our knife-wielding pathologist and her associates will be completely protected. Most research with less threatening viruses like the standard influenza strains is done by trained personnel in secure, well equipped, but relatively "normal" BSL-2 laboratories. At a minimum, any analysis of live pathogens that involves open containers requires access to glass-fronted, stainless-steel biohazard hoods where filtered (to remove viruses and bacteria) air blows onto the enclosed "bench top" and provides an "air curtain" at the open (generally 10–15 cm or so) interface.

In addition, the scientist/technician will be wearing disposable gloves and a dedicated laboratory gown (or coverall) that, depending on the level of security, will either remain permanently in the laboratory or will be discarded after use. All working surfaces will be wiped down with disinfectant. Contaminated "waste," "dirty bottles," and so forth may be dumped into disinfectant (hypochlorite solution) and/or later autoclaved (high pressure steam at +120°C for at least 15–20 minutes). Stainless steel is easy to clean, and entire laboratories are decontaminated by letting off a formaldehyde "bomb." That involves exiting fast and taping the doors after adding potassium permanganate ($KMnO_4$) to formalin—a solution of formaldehyde (CH_2O) in water—to releases the toxic gas. The lab is then abandoned for 24 hours, and only reentered after exhaust fans have cleared the air.

Beyond that "biosafety level 2" (BSL-2), dangerous pathogens are handled in negative pressure rooms and sealed hoods with glove ports, for BSL-3 to 3+ or, ultimately BSL-4, where the investigator is in a full "space-suit" with its own pumped air supply. On completing the task at hand, the BSL-3+ and BSL-4 scientists wash down with disinfectant, remove their protective gear and "shower-out" before changing back into street clothes. In the main, they are the only organisms that exit such a facility alive. All other materials are autoclaved-out and/or incinerated. Everything is done to minimize the possibility that the scientist could become infected, then pass some dangerous virus on to others.

Though it is not possible, at least under normal circumstances, to mandate that investigators who study the most dangerous human pathogens dwell apart from other people in monastic seclusion, those who research highly contagious virus infections of domestically important animals may, for example, be prohibited from living on a farm or having any contact with livestock. It takes a special type of person, with a high level of dedication, to work regularly under BSL-3+/BSL-4 level conditions. Also, the need to operate in such a cumbersome and expensive way can inhibit the progress of research on human pathogens. Most scientists are basically interested in ideas, and they will choose to work with systems that allow them to probe important issues without bothering too much about ultra-high security and excessive scrutiny.

How does infection happen?

In order to cause disease, viruses and bacteria must gain access to our body tissues, to enter what the great French physiologist Claude Bernard (1813–1878) termed the *milieu interieur*, the intracellular and extracellular spaces of our various organ systems. The basic requirement is that the invader must fulfill the necessary requirement for horizontal infection by traversing, or breaching, one or other of the cellular barriers that separate us from the external environment, namely the skin or the mucosal surfaces that line the gastrointestinal (GI) and respiratory tracts, the female reproductive tract, and the inner aspects of our various body orifices.

The skin, with a multilayered epidermis composed of flat squamous epithelium, a deeper layer of keratinocytes, then the thick, underlying dermis, is generally a tough protective barrier. The dermis contains resident host response cells, particularly the macrophages (big eaters) and another specialized category of skin phagocytes called Langerhans' cells that can act rapidly to engulf, and often destroy, any virus or bacterium that may enter through a skin abrasion. Once fed, these localized phagocytes can detach and travel in the lymph-containing lymphatics to the regional lymph nodes—we'll say more about them later—which is how Edward Jenner's scarified cowpox virus moved from a skin scratch to turn on a protective immune response in young James Phipps—and in hundreds of millions of people over the subsequent 200 years.

The lymphatics comprise a second circulation that drains extracellular fluid (lymph) from body tissues to return, via the "filter" of the lymphoid tissue, to our bloodstreams. Should this lymph flow be blocked mechanically by, for instance, large numbers of the mosquito-transmitted filarial parasite *Wucheraria bancrofti* accumulating in the lymphatics of the lower limbs, people suffer the gross leg swelling called elephantiasis. The dependent ankle thickening that most experience with advanced age is a sign of progressive heart failure and diminished activity: lymph return is a passive process that depends on the pumping action of exercised muscle groups.

As we have all experienced directly at one time or other, the skin is readily bypassed by some penetrating trauma that drives through to the deeper tissues. The best-case scenario is, of course, being jabbed through previously disinfected skin with a pristine hypodermic needle—a technology not available to Jenner—that delivers a protective vaccine, or a potentially lifesaving antibiotic, to the muscle below. Hypodermics were developed for this purpose, and it is part of the human tragedy that they are also used irresponsibly in ways that cause life-threatening diseases. Then there's the risk of localized bacterial infection when the trauma is caused by a rusty nail, knife stab, bullet wound, or, less immediately alarming though perhaps ultimately more dangerous, by the inserted proboscis of a virus-carrying mosquito or the biting mouth parts of an African tsetse fly carrying the trypanosome that causes sleeping sickness. We can generally limit our exposure to biting or stinging insects by wearing appropriate clothing and using chemical repellents. Most will avoid conflict zones if given the opportunity, though that's not necessarily true for places where people are consuming large amounts of alcohol. And wars are wars, not pandemics, though, like passive heart failure with age, they reflect characteristics endemic to the human condition.

While not as obviously "outside" as the skin, the "lumen," or inner, open (luminal) cavities of tubular organs like the gut, respiratory, and female reproductive tracts are also, at least in some senses, external to the body, or *milieu interieur*. All such surfaces are lined by what is called mucosal epithelium, or the mucosae. Again drained deeply to the lymph nodes via the lymphatics, the environment-exposed, outer cell layer of the mucosae is bathed in a protective layer of mucus, or slime. Secreted by specialized goblet cells, the mucin glycoprotein that dissolves in water is the basic component of mucus. Apart from mucin, mucus also contains a spectrum of salts and complex molecules, including natural antiseptics like the enzyme lysozyme and, in immune individuals, antibodies that are specific for potential pathogens. Mucus is also produced as saliva and tears. Should the mucus system go wrong, as it does in the human genetic disease cystic fibrosis that causes severe respiratory problems, the skin sweat glands that both excrete toxins and function as an important cooling mechanism when we are febrile (due to infection), or find ourselves in hot places, are also compromised.

The upper regions of the respiratory and GI tracts are generally similar, at least for anything that we take in by mouth. When it comes to the GI tract, though, the acid environment of the stomach tends to kill off many of the potential pathogens that we ingest, preventing their access to the intestines and below. Obviously, there is no similar mechanism to protect the fragile lung. Also, by limiting our food and fluid intake in discerning ways, by washing our hands before dining and by using utensils like knives, forks, and spoons, we minimize the risk that we will contract some infection via the GI tract. Hand hygiene is important, and we should minimize practices like picking our nose. I found the following on a website entitled "The Poetry of Sleazy Songs and Rotten Rhymes":

Yellow belly custard, Green snot pie. Mix it all together with a dead dogs eye. Slap it in a bucket nice 'n thick. Then wash it all down with a cup o' cold sick.

Nauseating, and definitely to be avoided and avoidable. But, apart from keeping our hands away from our face and maintaining a distance from those who are coughing and sneezing, it's much harder to avoid any contact with respiratory viruses than with GI tract, or enteric, pathogen.

Breathing is not optional. Asleep or awake, every hour of the day and night, we must breathe. The sole physiological exception is when we were fetuses living on oxygen (O_2) supplied by our mother's red blood cells (RBCs), via the placenta and umbilical cord, to the RBCs of the developing embryo. The reverse of this pathway gets rid of the excess carbon dioxide (CO_2) produced as a consequence of the normal processes of cell/tissue metabolism. After birth, we need to inspire and expire some 15–20 times a minute (for a normal adult at rest), or 50 times per minute at peak exercise. And we usually can't choose where to breathe.

Unless we're breathing through a respirator attached to a certified air or oxygen cylinder, or inhabit an enclosed, protected space, such as a pristine manufacturing facility (for electronics or nanotechnology) or a biosecurity research laboratory, where the incoming air is filtered, there's no guarantee anywhere that the atmosphere is clean. That's true even when we might assume that we are breathing fresh air. Facing the open ocean with a strong breeze coming off the sea would seem to be pretty safe, indeed bracing, but there's also an outside chance that dust from a big pile of lead-containing ore on a wharf area sited just around the picturesque headland (as occurred at Esperance in Western Australia) is just "blowin' in the wind."

The risk of transmission is minimized when we don't spit and take care to avoid the expulsion of infected aerosols (fluid droplets in air) by covering the mouth and nose with a handkerchief or tissue. If our hands are contaminated, we may transmit the infection to surfaces—called "fomites" by the epidemiologists—that are touched by others. Practicing cough etiquette is essential, especially when it comes to the education of children, who are often the primary source of a respiratory infection in any family. Hospitalizations in the United Kingdom during the influenza pandemic of 2009 showed two peaks, with a deep "valley" between them. The fall-off coincided exactly with the long summer vacation from school.

An unprotected cough generates a surprisingly large cloud of fine, aerosolized mucus. And the same thing happens, though to a much diminished extent, when we speak and even breathe.

The only thing that will ultimately stop respiratory spread is isolation of the infected individual. That's why, in most parts of the world—particularly the wealthier countries where the water and food supply is likely to be clean—severe respiratory infections are far and away the most likely to have serious, and even fatal, consequences. In addition, while it's possible to support a patient through, say, severe diarrhea, by fluid therapy, clearing a blocked-up lung is much more medically challenging.

What is snot?

Basically, snot and phlegm are mucus plus junk. The brush-like cilia on the surface of respiratory tract mucosal epithelial cells move mucus up and out. When we have an infection, our mucus is loaded with extras like "effete" (or dead) host response cells, bugs, all sorts of cell breakdown products, and so forth. Green or bright yellow snot likely reflects bacterial involvement. What we sneeze into our handkerchief or tissue could come just from the nose if, for example, the infection is caused by a common cold rhinovirus that doesn't spread further down the respiratory tract. Phlegm might be coughed up from deep in an influenza virus-infected lung. This stuff has to be cleared or it blocks the airways. At the other end of the body, mucus-laden fecal content can give way to the much more fluid, "pipe-stem" diarrhea that we associate with dysentery. The relative absence of mucus reflects that the pathogen has caused massive epithelial damage, while the loss of body water can kill by simple dehydration.

What is a horizontal infection? Is there another kind?

Most of the infections that we contract directly from other humans or from animals pass horizontally, that is, from donor X to recipient Y via contact with respiratory droplets (known as "aerosols"); saliva; or GI tract content containing viruses (influenza, rotavirus, hepatitis A virus) or bacteria (whooping cough). Others are transmitted horizontally by injection perhaps, in the past, on an unsterilized, hepatitis C virus-contaminated hypodermic needle, or at any time via the proboscis of a biting mosquito or tick that is infected with one or other arthropod-borne virus (arbovirus). Some pathogens are generally less infectious. That's true of HIV/AIDS, which only transmits as a consequence of vaginal or anal sex, or following exposure to contaminated blood. All pandemic infections are basically horizontal in character.

Vertical transmission occurs when a pathogen goes directly from mother to child. That can happen when a virus such as measles or rubella (German measles) passes through the layers of the placenta to infect the fetus. The *in utero* transmission of viruses like rubella or cytomegalovirus (CMV) can lead to premature termination. Should the fetus not abort, the consequences for a surviving infant may—depending on the developmental stage when the exposure occurs—be a spectrum of abnormalities ranging from microcephaly (small brain) to eye cataracts, to learning and psychological problems in children who may seem relatively normal at birth. Every adult woman of childbearing age should ensure that she is vaccinated against measles, mumps, and rubella before becoming pregnant. Regrettably, we don't yet have a CMV vaccine.

With regard to a newborn baby, the mucus membranes of the infant may be exposed to contaminated blood at parturition if the mother has some persistent infection. Also, the ingestion of virus-containing breast milk and (in some cultures) saliva-contaminated, pre-masticated food can spread HIV/AIDS. In this case, steps are taken to prevent such horizontal transmission by ensuring that any HIV-positive, pre-parturient (or nursing) mother is receiving anti-viral drugs.

Are all virus and bacterial infections bad for us?

It depends on the type of infection. Not all the microorganisms that live in, or on, us are potential pathogens. Some, described generally as commensals, survive happily on the luminal sur-faces of the mucosal epithelia that line the respiratory and GI tracts. The bacteria that inhabit the human intestines produce both enzymes (which help break down various foodstuffs) and essential nutrients like vitamin B7 (biotin), vitamin B12, and niacin. The normal GI, or gut, bacterial flora makes up about 50% of human fecal dry mass and, apart from the contribution to diet, also denies "space" to other, more pathogenic micro-organisms. Recently, there has been a great deal of interest in defining what constitutes this healthy "microbiome," particu-larly from the aspect that excessive antibiotic treatment may skew these GI tract bacterial populations to favor colonization by "bad bugs," which might, for instance, produce toxins that are absorbed across the wall of the gut into our bloodstream.

Commensal microorganisms may not, however, be totally friendly. Normally benign GI tract and respiratory tract resi-dents like *Cryptosporidium* (a protozoan) and *Pneumocystis* (a fungus) can invade our tissues to cause, respectively, poten-tially fatal diarrhea or respiratory problems when our protec-tive immune systems fail as a consequence of, for example, the massive immunosuppression that can result from cancer therapy, or the almost inevitable immune collapse in untreated (with drugs) patients infected with the HIV/AIDS virus. Most of us experience a permanent association with the bacterium *Staphylococcus aureus*, which lives on our skin, causes boils and pimples from time to time, and can be a major problem follow-ing surgery. Even so, while commensal organisms can become pathogenic in compromised individuals and are sometimes responsible for dangerous hospital outbreaks (golden Staph), these never cause epidemics, let alone pandemics.

If there is a bacterial and protozoal "microbiome," is there also a "virome"?

Yes, we all have a "virome," and the viruses that we carry through life in our body tissues are sometimes far from benign. Prominent in this regard are the large DNA herpes-viruses, including cytomegalovirus (CMV), *Herpes simplex* (HSV)—HSV1 causes cold sores and HSV2 reproductive tract infections—*Herpes zoster* (chicken pox in the young, shingles in the elderly), and Epstein Barr virus (EBV). Some (*H.simplex* and *H.zoster*) go latent, or hide out, in the bodies of different nerve cells, then reactivate to cause local damage to the lip, mucosae, or skin. Others, particularly EBV, can cause various forms of cancer. You will read more about these when we discuss HIV/AIDS.

Mostly, though it is of no obvious benefit to us, we live in reasonable accommodation with our virome and, while recurrent HSV2 can be very debilitating, these unwanted passengers in our tissues rarely reactivate to cause lethal disease. We will discuss some exceptions later when talking about the AIDS problem. And, unless they mutate to spread via aerosol transmission, the familiar human herpesviruses are very unlikely to cause pandemics. The probability of any such change may be infinitesimal, though it is the case that a distant relative causes the respiratory problem infectious laryngotracheitis in chickens. Also, Marek's disease (a herpesvirus-induced inflammatory neuropathy) transmits when birds breathe in cellular material shed from infected feather follicles. Both viruses are endemic globally and, as they are major problems for chicken producers, there are vaccines.

Also, while most herpesviruses have a very limited host range, the *H. simplex*–like virus (*Herpesvirus simiae*, or B virus) that forms part of the rhesus macaque virome has caused severe encephalitis (20–26 cases, with 16 deaths) in animal handlers and scientists who study non-human primates. The latest to die (in 1997) was researcher Elizabeth Griffin, as a consequence of being splashed in the eye while working at the Yerkes National Primate Center in Atlanta. There could be other viruses like that out there in some wildlife reservoir.

Returning to the virome: our feces also contain the genetic signatures of viruses that we happen to have ingested in food, or are bacteriophages living in our gut microbiome. As discussed above, all organisms have their own spectra of infecting viruses. Some are lethal and some are harmless passengers. The plants we eat can contain viruses that, while doing us no harm, pass through our GI tracts. Groundwater contamination with human fecal material can, for example, be monitored by testing for the genome of the plant pathogen pepper mild mottle virus, which has been ingested at one end of our GI tract to emerge (at least as surviving viral RNA) at the other. Think about that the next time you enjoy a salad with sliced bell pepper!

What does "immunity" mean?

Immunity (my research field) is very complicated, and the main focus here will be to get across a few points that may help you to understand both what happens when a bad infection comes along and what we might do to prevent, or ameliorate, such a situation. The word "immunity" comes from the Latin *immunis*, meaning "without tax." Members of the *genio immunium* in Imperial Rome were legionnaires who enjoyed a tax-exempt status after returning from the wars and/or garrison duty to maintain the Empire. They pledged allegiance to Minerva, the Roman goddess of wisdom and war. With her distinctive coat of mail, helmet, and spear, Minerva provides a symbol of leadership and intellect that is widely used by contemporary institutions. She could also be thought of as symbolizing the protection conferred by immunity, together with the wisdom of vaccinating both our children and ourselves.

The vertebrate immune system has in fact evolved to minimize the tax of parasitism by simple agents that reproduce, and thus change more quickly, than us: the viruses, bacteria, protozoa, and other pathogens. It must be ready for anything that nature throws at us and, with a lot of help from sanitation, antibiotics, vaccines, and the like in recent times, it generally does a spectacularly good job. The true foot soldiers and warriors of immunity, particularly the white blood cells (WBCs) and their products, live within us and have been around in biology for hundreds of millions of years.

The broad-spectrum, innate immune response that cuts in immediately when we are first infected utilizes mechanisms like phagocytosis (engulfment, followed by destruction in toxic, sub-cellular organelles) that are ubiquitous in biology, with some elements being represented in species as evolutionarily distant as fruit flies and us. The very specific adaptive immune response that we prime by vaccination is unique to the vertebrates and is found only in the jawed fish and species above on the evolutionary ladder. Adaptive immunity is thought to have arrived with a "big bang" about 350–400 million years back. Of course, that "big bang" could have lasted for a million or more years, but we have no way of probing the issue. Overall, the innate and adaptive and immune systems work together to promote an optimal host response.

The first thing that happens when we are infected with a pathogen is that the invading virus or bacterium triggers an innate response on the part of parasitized—and neighboring—cells that is largely mediated via secreted molecules called cytokines and chemokines. The type 1 interferons, for example, are cytokine proteins that function to limit the early phases of growth for some viruses (especially influenza), while the defensins are peptides that hold bacteria in check. In addition, the cytokines and chemokines provide signals that induce various categories of circulating WBCs to exit into the compromised tissues and/or organs via the blood vessel walls. These innate-response WBCs, all of which are produced in the bone marrow, include the neutrophils (also called granulocytes), monocytes, and macrophages that act to phagocytose and destroy invading bacteria and/or virus-damaged cells and, in turn, produce more cytokines and chemokines.

Spilling over into the blood, the cytokines also act as endogenous pyrogens, which operate to perturb the temperature-setting mechanism in the hypothalamus and induce fever.

Along with the fact that some cytokines can further target other parts of the brain to make us drowsy, being febrile (hot) causes us to feel bad, and we slow down. This is one situation where we should be respectful of what our body is telling us and take it easy. In addition, fever limits the replication of those viruses and bacteria that prefer to grow at lower temperatures. High fever can be life threatening if it goes on for too long, but it is generally a protective mechanism.

Without this early innate response to hold infections in check, the body could quickly be overwhelmed by, for instance, a rapidly growing bacterial pathogen, a condition referred to as septicemia. The downside is, though, that the innate response can be over-effulgent and the patient suffers a condition called cytokine shock. What is thought to happen in some forms of hi-path influenza infection, for instance, is that the toxic side effects of particular host response molecules result in massive vascular leakage, with the consequence that patients effectively drown in their own lung fluids. This is poorly understood, and much current research is focused on dissecting the underlying mechanisms so that pharmacologists and physicians can develop appropriate therapeutic strategies.

While innate immunity can slow down the progress of the infection, it is generally a blunt instrument that does not have the capacity to eliminate the invader. That is the role of the more slowly developing adaptive immune response. Adaptive immunity is a property of other WBCs, the B and T lymphocytes. Its effectiveness depends on the enormous diversity of the B cell and T cell receptor (TCR) repertoires that react, in the main, to the presence of foreign invaders.

The T cells, or T lymphocytes, develop in the thymus gland in our neck so that each individual cell (or clonal precursor) expresses multiple copies of a single-specificity TCR molecule that, while not reacting to our own body tissues (a protective mechanism called self-tolerance), is programmed to recognize "altered-self" proteins on the surface of other cells. I won't go into the details of the "altered-self" story—which is what earned me and my Swiss colleague Rolf Zinkernagel a Nobel Prize—as it is very complicated and beyond what you need to deal with in the present context. At its simplest, the altered-self molecules are specialized proteins that form in the cell cytoplasm, then "pick up" a small bit (an 8–12 amino acid peptide) of a viral or bacterial protein and carry it to the surface of the infected cell. There it can be seen as "foreign" (or non-self) by the "best fit"—think lock and key—TCR on a roaming T cell.

With regard to the virus-specific T cells themselves, there are two main categories, characterized broadly as CD8+ T "killers"—or cytotoxic T lymphocytes (CTLs)—and CD4+ T "helpers," each of which recognizes a different type of altered-self. The CD8+ CTLs, the "hit men" of immunity, are programmed to seek out and destroy all virus-infected cells that express the "cognate" (complementary to their TCR) altered-self. The CD4+ helpers, on the other hand, are particularly focused on altered-self complexes presented on the surface of "stimulator" dendritic cells that, subsequent to phagocytosis or endocytosis, process foreign proteins to give immunogenic (also called antigenic) peptide fragments. If you're wondering, CD stands for "cluster of differentiation," while 4 and 8 refer to different surface proteins that—after staining with fluorochrome-labeled monoclonal antibodies—allow us to separate these two categories of T lymphocytes.

Some 5 to 7 days prior to becoming a fully functional killer, the TCRs of a few naïve CD8+ CTL precursors will have encountered their "cognate altered-self" molecules on stimulator cells in the lymph node. If you don't know about lymph nodes, these are the "glands" in our neck, groin, and armpit that can swell up and become painful when we get an infection. These rare, small "ancestral" CD8+ T lymphocyte precursors then divide every 6 to 8 hours or so to give the numerous, large, activated CD8+ CTL effectors that ultimately exit and, following the trail laid by various chemokine/cytokine signals, make their way to other body tissues (lung for influenza, liver for hepatitis) where the virus is growing. There they get on with the job of "bumping off" infected cells. After the virus has been cleared, some CD8+ T cells remain in a "poised" memory state and can be induced to respond more rapidly if the same pathogen is encountered again. The CD4+ T "helpers," on the other hand, function principally by secreting cytokines (like interleukin 2 and interleukin 4) that, again in the lymph nodes, promote the division and differentiation of other immune cell types, including the B cells and CD8+ T cells. Also, in the case of infections caused by bacteria and by the big DNA viruses—like the herpesviruses discussed above—CD4+ T cell effectors that produce large amounts of the cytokine γ interferon invade into sites of infection, where they play a major part in controlling the pathogen.

But, while the CD8+ CTL and CD4+ helper T cell responses are important for bringing any infectious process to an end, it is the "humoral" immunity mediated via the B lymphocytes, or B cells, that is of greatest interest when it comes to protective vaccines. Why are these particular WBCs called B lymphocytes? In the chicken, which has an adaptive immune system that ultimately works much like our own, the B cells develop in a separate organ called the Bursa of Fabricius. This organ does not exist in mammals, where the site of B cell origin is the bone marrow. Every T cells and B cell shares the theme of expressing a very specific cell surface receptor, called TCR and immunoglobulin (Ig), respectively. The major difference is that the Ig+ B lymphocytes are not processed through the thymus, and Ig is not targeted to altered-self molecules, as is the TCR. Thus, while the TCR remains attached to the CD8+ killer or CD4+ helper, the B cells differentiate to give large, protein-producing plasma cells that pump out (secrete) masses of Ig (antibody) into tissue fluids and, ultimately, the blood. These free-floating antibodies will bind to—and thus facilitate the elimination of—any foreign protein (immunogen, or antigen); virus; or bacterium.

Furthermore, under the influence of cytokines produced by the CD4+ helper T cells, the immune B cells undergo a process called "class-switching" to give various antibody forms that can mediate somewhat different outcomes in immunity. In addition, CD4+ T help drives "affinity maturation," whereby "somatic mutation" leads to the emergence, through sequential cell division, of B cell/plasma cell clonotypes that produce higher affinity (better binding) antibodies. As with the TCRs, there are millions of different Ig specificities, ready for anything that the world of pathogens can bring forward to challenge us.

With regard to those class-switched Ig types, the IgG molecule is Y shaped, with identical specific binding sites on two of the arms that "grab hold" of the complementary (cognate again) viral antigen (protein) and "neutralize" the virus. The IgG "third arm" has a common region (Fc) that binds to receptors on cells like macrophages, leading to the engulfment (endocytosis, phagocytosis) and destruction of the antigen/ antibody complexes. Another Ig type is IgA, which can transit across mucosal surfaces and is especially important in gut and lung immunity. IgE, meanwhile, has evolved to expel worms but, as an unwanted side effect, can mistake substances like plant pollen for a worm and thus cause allergy.

Overall, the main difference between immune T cells and the antibodies produced by the B cell/plasma cells is thus that the secreted Ig molecules bind principally to proteins, whether in free form or on the surface of virus particles and bacteria, while the T lymphocytes are targeted to pathogen-modified cells. Furthermore, the fact that antibodies may circulate in the blood for life after a single exposure to a particular virus, bacterium, or vaccine means that they are readily detected using a spectrum of straightforward diagnostic tests that might, for example, involve the use of blood serum (the fluid phase) to neutralize virus infectivity for chick embryos or tissue cultures, or just measure serum Ig binding to a viral protein dried onto a plastic surface. Though, for instance, we did not understand the full identity of the 1918–1919 pandemic flu virus until it was resurrected 90 years after the event, we had known its basic H1N1 "serotype" for decades as a consequence of being able to detect the antibody "footprints" of that much earlier, and long gone, infection in the blood of survivors.

While both undoubtedly benefit from occasional boosting, perhaps by a further vaccine "shot" that induces cell division and increases numbers, clones of memory B cells and T cells have been shown to persist for five decades or more. The plasma cell "factories" sit for years in the bone marrow, where they continue to pump out their particular Ig molecule, and they may also "hang around" in the gut- and bronchus-associated lymphoid tissue (GALT and BALT, respectively) in the GI tract and the lung. The same is true for the "resting" memory CD4+ and CD8+ T cells that continue to "roam" the body long after the pathogen is eliminated. Furthermore, positive serum antibody tests do indeed correlate with protection. Those who still had circulating antibodies specific for the 1918 flu virus after being infected initially were resistant when a similar, though much milder, pathogen returned in 1977. Immune T cells, on the other hand, provide no immediate barrier to reinfection, as they must first be re-stimulated, generally in the lymph nodes, then divide and differentiate again to be CTL effectors. These "recall" responses can be massive and, as will be discussed later, may have a part to play as we seek to develop improved immunization strategies.

Viral vaccines, particularly the live, attenuated vaccines used to prevent infections like yellow fever, polio, measles, and mumps, cause very mild, transient, localized infections that function to induce the continued presence of CD4+ and CD8+ T cells and primed B cells/plasma cells. Protective antibodies continue to circulate in the blood, while memory T cells may be rapidly recalled to cell division and effector function when the individual later encounters the naturally spreading, and more virulent, "wild type" virus. In the case of someone who has been infected with HIV and, untreated with drugs, is on the road to developing AIDS, there's a catch-22 in that, during this process of cell proliferation and differentiation, "activated" CD4+ T cells responding to any invading organism are particularly susceptible to being infected with HIV. This contributes to the progressive decline in CD4+ T cell numbers, which leads ultimately to the development of full-blown AIDS.

Contact your doctor, or local sexually transmitted diseases clinic, immediately if you have even the slightest suspicion that you might have been exposed to HIV. Should that concern only come to the fore after, say, three weeks or more, there are now quick antibody tests that can be performed "on the spot" within 30 minutes. But don't wait!

I know that this is complicated stuff. If your head hurts after reading this, don't worry. Even a medical hematologist colleague told me that immunology was too much for him. There are just a few very simple points that you need to retain for our discussion of pandemics. The first is that, while we can't prime such mechanisms to enhance long-term protection, innate immunity is very important, even though it can also have deleterious consequences (cytokine shock) if it should come on too strongly. The second is that adaptive immunity is extraordinarily specific and, once primed, protective antibodies, memory B cells/plasma cells, and CD4+ and CD8+ T lymphocytes can stick around for decades, both as the "footprints" of a prior infection and to protect us against reinfection with the same, or a very closely related, organism. The third is that the antibodies, which bind principally to cell surface proteins on viruses and bacteria (or to secreted bacterial toxins), are the main line of defense put in place by vaccination, which is simply a process that, while in a much less damaging way, mimics infection.

What are monoclonal antibodies?

Monoclonal antibodies, the mAbs, revolutionized biology. As soon as immunologists realized that a single B lymphocyte (and its progeny plasma cell) produces just one type of very specific antibody (Ig) molecule, the race was on to grow such cells out in culture so that masses of the product, the fabulous mAbs, could be made. The problem was cracked in 1975 with the development of the hybridoma approach by University of Cambridge researchers Cesar Milstein (an Argentinian) and Georges Kohler (a German). Kohler and Milstein shared the 1984 Nobel Prize with Nils Jerne (a Dane), who made substantial contributions to our understanding of "background," or "natural" immunity.

At first, the main and massive consequence of the mAb technology for infectious disease research was to produce a range of defined probes specific for different viral and bacterial proteins, and for the variants that emerge following gene mutation. A further, major advance resulted from the fact that monospecific reagents to detect human proteins, for example, could now be readily made by immunizing mice with a particular cell type or tissue, then isolating a mouse hybridoma cell line secreting an mAb that is specific for the human molecule of interest. Apart from the obvious applications in research for, say, localizing particular proteins in tissues, this led to a whole new spectrum of better diagnostic tests.

As mentioned above, dividing human T lymphocytes into the CD4+ and CD8+ T cell compartments depends on the use of mouse mAbs conjugated to different fluorochromes, like fluorescein (FITC) and allophycocyanin (APC). Using a machine called a flow cytometer, such mAb-stained lymphocytes are dispersed in fluid and made to flow past a laser beam that induces green (for FITC) or red (for APC) fluorescence. Positive cells are counted and, if desired, "sorted" into separate streams to give defined populations. Sophisticated research flow cytometers use several lasers to stain for 12 or more such fluorochromes simultaneously, giving massive data sets that require heavy duty computing. In simpler mode, access to a very modest machine that can be found in minimally equipped "field" laboratories allows the diagnosis of AIDS to be made by calculating blood CD4+/CD8+ T cell ratios.

More recently, mAbs are increasingly being used in cancer therapy, and they are also being produced to protect against a spectrum of infectious challenges. Perhaps the first major therapeutic/protective application in human disease has been to substitute mAbs for pooled human serum Ig to protect very young babies against infection with respiratory syncytial virus. Also, given that injected mAbs persist in the blood for much longer than most drugs, some researchers and practical technologists are focusing on the possibility that they could be produced rapidly in large quantities to protect front-line personnel, like immigration officials, health care workers, police, and so forth in the face of, say, an emerging influenza pandemic.

Would you describe mAbs as drugs or vaccines?

We tend to refer to mAbs as "biologicals." The principle is the same as giving a drug in the sense that both are made outside the body and are injected into someone, though only drugs are likely to be taken by mouth. Obviously, an injected (or absorbed) chemical or protein (mAb) only has an effect for as long as it persists in our blood and/or organs. All such substances are ultimately cleared (excreted) or metabolized (consumed or changed). Drugs are chemicals, or mixes of chemicals, made synthetically (small molecules like aspirin and ibuprofen) or by a plant (the cancer drug Taxol). A vaccine, on the other hand, mimics an infection and stimulates the immune response to produce clonally expanded B cells/plasma cells, and thus protective antibodies, in the very long term.

With the mAbs, the last thing we want is for them to act as a vaccine. The body may see the injected mAb as "foreign" and make an immune response against it. Then, if used for a second round of treatment, they will be recognized by, in effect, anti-antibodies (called anti-idiotypic antibodies) and eliminated immediately. That's why it's important to use human (rather than mouse) mAbs for therapy and/or prophylaxis (prevention). The mouse proteins are more "foreign" and thus likely to trigger an immune response. The mAbs clearly have a place in the armory of infectious disease physicians with, for example, a recent research paper describing the production of mAbs that protect against both the influenza A and B viruses that we discuss in more detail later.

What are vaccines?

To briefly summarize, a vaccine itself might be an attenuated, or weakened, virus that doesn't multiply much; a "killed" product—influenza virus grown in eggs and then inactivated to a non-infectious form with formalin; or a single virus surface protein made by recombinant DNA technology. There are also "virus-like particles" used, for example, in the anti-papilloma virus vaccine, that are, again, non-living and non-infectious.

The non-living vaccines will generally be injected with some form of adjuvant, a substance that—by inducing the secretion of chemokines/cytokines and the like—cries "danger" to the immune system and tells it to get going. Commonly used adjuvants are the chemical alum (hydrated aluminum sulfates) and various oils and synthetic substances. A great deal of current research is focused on exploring the adjuvant potential of proteins that are involved in normal innate immune responses. Some argue that the only solution to the tuberculosis (TB) problem, for example, is to produce an effective vaccine. That would be a major triumph. Using a "whole bug" (killed or attenuated) TB vaccine approach would have the advantage that some TB lipoproteins—protein plus fat, like the cholesterol transporters in our blood—are great adjuvants. Then the organism is so big that we could potentially add (by inserting the DNA) a whole lot of molecules from other viruses and bacteria to make a "one shot" product.

Most vaccines are (as with mAbs) injected, but kids take the live Sabin polio vaccine by mouth on a sugar lump, or inhale the live *Flumist* to prevent influenza. There is a difference between live and killed or inactivated vaccines in that only the live products actually infect cells and stimulate the CD8+ CTL response. The proteins in killed vaccines are phagocytosed at the site of injection by macrophages, particularly the dendritic cell variety that stimulates the CD4+ helper T cells, and are carried (as described earlier in this section) to the lymph nodes in the blood or lymph to trigger an immune response.

Apart from the fact that a vaccine doesn't make you sick (though, because of the cytokines and chemokines, it can give you a sore arm and transient fever), the big advantage of being immunized (and having protective antibodies) is that you stop an incoming virus from damaging large numbers of your cells and going all through your body to hang out in some site "protected" from the immune system. There's a suggestion at the moment that West Nile virus (WNV) may sometimes hide in the kidney to give progressive renal pathology. The bacterial disease leptospirosis is characterized by long-term persistence and continued replication in the kidney tubules, even though the infected person or animal has made a vigorous immune response against this invading spirochete. Fortunately, that can be cleared out by treatment with an antibiotic such as streptomycin ("strepto for lepto"). We discuss TB, WNV, and leptospirosis later. With regard to childhood vaccination, I believe that dealing with a whiny or grumpy kid for a couple of days is a much better option than permanent damage (such as chronic lung or brain problems) or death from some hideous pathogen.

2

PANDEMICS, EPIDEMICS, AND OUTBREAKS

What is the exact definition of pandemic?

A novel infection—new and previously unconfronted—that spreads globally and results in a high incidence of morbidity (sickness) and mortality (death) has, for the past 300 years or more, been described as a "pandemic." The word derives from *pan*—"across"—and *demos*, meaning "people" or "population." A pandemic spreads across all people. The 1918–1919 flu virus disseminated worldwide, without regard to race, location, cultural belief system, or social status.

There is, though, some disagreement about how and when the term should be used. Until very recently, evidence of contagion monitored by the rapid spread of unfamiliar and generally distressing symptoms was still the main measure of a new, readily transmitted disease. Before the germ theory of infection became established in the mid- to late nineteenth century and for many years thereafter, the prevalence and severity of clinical impairment was all that we had to go on. As summarized in the previous chapter, that situation has now vastly changed, with the 150-year—and continuing—progression in the unraveling of infectious diseases and the incredible advances in both understanding and diagnostic technology that advanced gradually until the 1980s or so, to gather ever increasing momentum with the molecular biology revolution of the past 30 years. Now, modern science provides us with tests that enable the identification of any causative organism both quickly and definitively.

This capacity for rapid diagnosis means that we no longer rely solely, if at all, on seeing severe symptoms. A readily detectable infectious agent that, like the 2009 SW flu virus, tends to cause relatively mild disease in most people but spreads rapidly around the planet will, according to currently used criteria, legitimately be described as causing a pandemic. That's where confusion can arise: the general sense is that "pandemic" is synonymous with catastrophe. With both the media and the broader population ultimately perceiving that the 2009 SW flu pandemic was no more dangerous than the familiar, recurring, "seasonal" influenza epidemics, many had the sense that the regulatory and public health authorities had vastly overstated the level of risk.

Who declares a pandemic?

Pandemic infections are, by definition, global problems that cannot be dealt with exclusively by individual nation-states. Epidemiologists, statisticians, and other professionals working at the World Health Organization (WHO) based in Geneva, Switzerland, have the responsibility for declaring whether or not a pandemic is occurring. Charged with monitoring and protecting human health everywhere on the planet, the WHO is one of the better functioning agencies of the United Nations. Unlike some UN operations, it rarely attracts the ire of political extremists and xenophobes. Even so, the June 11, 2009, WHO decision to raise the level of influenza pandemic alert from Phase 5 to Phase 6 ultimately stimulated a great deal of negative media commentary. This first flu pandemic of the twenty-first century just wasn't up to expectations!

Nonetheless, working with various national bodies, the WHO generally does a good job, and the 2009 influenza experience illustrates the various stages that culminate in the declaration of a pandemic.

Was the H1N1 "swine flu" really so mild?

It gets a mixed review. Part of the perception that the 2009 H1N1 SW flu was not so bad reflects that those in the 65+ age groups, who are usually the most vulnerable in a typical influenza epidemic, were relatively unaffected due to protective immunity acquired by exposure to a cross-reactive virus that had since disappeared from human populations. As we discussed in the previous chapter, immune memory can last for 50, even for 70 or more years. On the other side of good/bad equation for the 2009 virus was the evidence of more severe disease and a greater incidence of hospitalization in indigenous communities than is usually seen with influenza. This could be a reflection of poor background health due to diabetes, malnutrition, alcoholism, and so forth, but there are also some indications of a genetic susceptibility component.

In addition, when compared with the normal "seasonal" flu strains, the admission of pregnant women in the third trimester to critical care beds was very high, and it seemed to affect a disproportionate number of fit, young adults. Some were saved by being hooked up to an ECMO (extra corporeal membrane oxygenation) machine that effectively rested their lungs during the process of natural repair. While 50% of those who would likely have died without ECMO made a full recovery, this is a scarce, expensive technology, and along with the available critical care beds, that emergency resource was quickly overwhelmed. The normal load of, for example, pediatric cardiac repair operations had to be cancelled until the emergency was over.

In reality, the WHO was not doing so badly when it called the 2009 influenza a pandemic. Though the WHO (like any global operation, public or private) has its limitations, only an international organization can (with the help of national agencies) take the ultimate responsibility for declaring that humanity is facing a pandemic. That has to be done with care and must follow established guidelines. The rules have to be clearly thought through and stated, as the ensuing response will require the deployment of substantial administrative and physical resources. Sounding the pandemic alarm can't simply be left to the ad hoc judgment of a select few key individuals, no matter how wise and well-informed they may be. The turnover rate for WHO officials can be high and even mandatory, given strict rules governing the duration of contracts, retirement at age 60, and so forth. Being part of a global agency, WHO officers may also come from very different cultural and economic backgrounds. What ranks as common sense for one particular group may seem less clear for others.

How does the WHO operate?

While the central office is in Geneva, the planet is divided for administrative purposes into 6 regions: Africa, Europe, the Eastern Mediterranean, Southeast Asia, the Western Pacific, and the Americas. Each has a WHO office that serves between 11 and 53 different countries and, as can be seen in Figure 2.1, the division is not strictly geographic. The Regional Office for the Western Pacific, which includes nations as diverse in geography, size, and location as Australia, China, and Tuvalu, is located in Manila, while that for Southeast Asia is in New Delhi. Some Indonesian territories located, for example, to the west of China on a standard global map come under the Southeast Asia office.

With influenza, the WHO defines six grades of *Pandemic Alert Phase,* based on the incidence of the disease and the extent of spread within and between the various regions. The criteria are published and available on the Web for all to see. A *Phase 2 Alert,* for example, merely informs public health officials, the

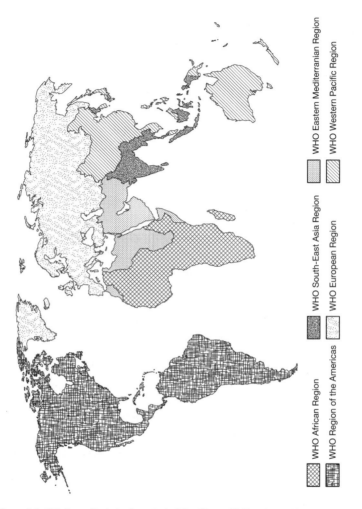

Figure 2.1. This figure illustrates the extent of the different WHO regions, which relate to the location of the WHO regional offices, rather than to any strict geographic division of the planet. The fact that a Phase 6 Pandemic Alert is issued when a novel, rapidly spreading influenza A virus is found to cause disease in more than one region illustrates how, if that criterion is used, a pandemic could be legitimately declared for, say, a mosquito-borne pathogen (like the Chikungunya alphavirus) that is expanding its territorial impact while still operating within the confines of one continental land mass. Chikungunya, which comes out of Africa, has in fact already extended beyond that range by moving around the Indian Ocean rim, down into Indonesia and Irian Jaya, and up into Italy.

Reproduced with permission from the World Health Organization.

media, and anyone who cares to look that a new influenza virus has emerged from some animal reservoir (such as pigs, in the case of the 2009 pandemic) and is causing infection in people. *Phase 4* means that human-to-human transmission is at a level where there is a continuing, sustainable outbreak within a community. *Phase 5* means that the outbreak has now spread to at least two countries in a particular WHO region. The final *Phase 6 Alert* is issued when human-to-human spread progresses from one WHO region to a second and significant numbers of people are infected.

This classification system, which depends on the distribution and prevalence of the infection, means that the declaration of a *Phase 6* influenza pandemic alert does not basically depend on the virulence, or pathogenicity, of the particular influenza A virus. But, given that the terms "pandemic" and "catastrophe" are synonymous to most people, why not change the definition? The problem is that doing so means coupling two different criteria and deciding ahead of time on outcomes that may not ultimately prove to be valid. For example, an influenza infection that seems to be not too bad when it occurs among those who are adequately housed and fed in a wealthy country may prove to be a true catastrophe for the less fortunate. Differences between rich and poor nations involve more than food and shelter, and include a multitude of factors like the availability of medical oxygen support and rapid access to the appropriate antibiotics for treating secondary bacterial infections that can deliver the *coup de grace* in a viral pneumonia.

Then, apart from any social disadvantage, there is the genetic variation that can distinguish ethnic groups and the threat, particularly with influenza, that the virus may mutate to a more virulent form. "Pandemic" applies to all populations equally, even when they are not in fact equal. Once a novel pathogen starts to spread rapidly and widely, a pandemic must be declared.

Should the pandemic classification system be refined?

There are many who think so. One possibility would be to have it reflect two numbers: the first denoting how bad a disease is clinically, and the second the extent of transmission. Thus, we might describe a generally mild but highly transmissible disease as a Level 2/6 pandemic—low clinical profile but high potential of transmission. That would pretty much characterize what happened in 2009 with the H1N1 SW flu, while the 1918–1919 influenza might have been a 5/6. Why 5/6 and not 6/6? Well, it doesn't look to have been as severe overall as the greater than 50% mortality associated with the relatively small number (less than 600 so far) of cases caused by the H5N1 "bird flu" virus. There is, though, some discussion that, because these H5N1 viruses (and the vaccines made from them) tend to stimulate suboptimal antibody responses in humans, the background infection rates may have been greatly underestimated, at least in those Asian communities where there is the possibility of widespread contact with infected domestic ducks, quail, and chickens.

The only time we might have seen anything like a "6/6" severity in humans during recorded history was the successive outbreaks of plague in medieval Europe. The worst possible "fast" 6/6 scenario is the hypothetical disease portrayed in the movie *Contagion*, where just about everyone who is infected seems to die horribly and the virus transmits with extraordinary ease. The fact that in the absence of drug treatment HIV/AIDS eventually kills almost everyone it infects would make it a "slow" 6/1 if we just rely on numbers and count all members of the community, rather than limiting our survey to those who are sexually active, are injecting drug users, or happen to be born to an untreated HIV carrier. On the other hand, if we accept the influenza criteria for extension to different regions, HIV could also be described as a "slow" 6/6 pandemic. With regard to AIDS, the WHO did not make a big deal about declaring a pandemic alert. That would have been pointless, as the disease had been so widely publicized over the 6 years from the time the first cases were diagnosed in New York and California until the 1987 launch of the Global Program on AIDS. The AIDS pandemic is now in its third or, perhaps, its fourth decade, but who would quibble about the difference?

How does a pandemic differ from an epidemic or an outbreak?

These different categorizations are somewhat arbitrary, as they depend both on the novelty of a particular infection and the extent of global spread. As discussed in more detail in the later chapter on influenza, an "immune-escape" variant of an influenza A virus strain that has been circulating for years in human populations and spreads worldwide is said to be causing a "seasonal epidemic," while a new virus that has emerged from some animal reservoir (pigs in 2009) is described as a pandemic pathogen. In subsequent chapters, some of the infections we will consider have to date caused little more than very limited, geographically constrained outbreaks. Even so, chance often plays a considerable part in determining the spectrum of what actually happens, so telling the stories of these "experiments of nature" provides insights into potential, future pandemics.

Every pandemic begins as a perhaps unrecognized outbreak that in turn leads to an epidemic. Again, it's a matter of novelty and transmission. A prominent example of a disease that emerged suddenly from a wildlife reservoir is the 2002 severe acute respiratory syndrome (SARS). It began as an outbreak, became an epidemic, and at least as far as the U.S. Centers for Disease Control and Prevention (CDC) were concerned, was the first pandemic of the twenty-first century. It certainly fulfilled the WHO's *Phase 5 Influenza Alert* criterion by spreading between humans in more than two countries in a WHO region (Western Pacific: China, Singapore, Vietnam) and then crossed the final *Phase 6 Alert* bridge by transmitting to, and causing further cases in, a second region: Toronto in the Americas. But, while SARS was also carried to other nations (including

Australia and the United States) by infected travelers, there was no additional (or secondary) spread to colleagues, family members, or medical personnel. In the following chapter, we discuss what did happen with SARS in more detail, and you will realize that this was purely a matter of chance. The difference between SARS and the 2009 influenza pandemic was that, though both were caused by novel viruses, the number of SARS cases remained relatively small throughout. That's where SARS may fail the WHO's pandemic test.

There's no doubt that SARS would, however, satisfy the criteria for traditional and sometimes historic terms like "plagues" and "pestilences" that have much the same connotation as "epidemic" or "pandemic." The term "plague" is used both in a generic sense, to characterize any widespread infection, and to describe the plague, the terrible systemic disease caused by the bacterium *Yersinia pestis* that is normally maintained in a rodent (rat, mouse, squirrel)–flea (*Xenopsylla cheopsis*) transmission cycle. In the absence of any understanding of the cause, *Y. pestis* caused recurrent outbreaks and epidemics that killed millions of people in fourteenth to eighteenth-century Europe. A classical zoonosis, the severe respiratory form (pneumonic plague) can sometimes be associated with human-to-human spread. Such outbreaks occur occasionally in India, and *Y. pestis* was used as a biological warfare agent in World War II. Now, if caught early, it can be readily treated with standard antibiotics like streptomycin and tetracycline.

"Pestilence" has tended to fall out of modern usage, and it is most often encountered within a medieval or religious context (and perhaps the occasional heavy metal band). In Albrecht Durer's *Four Horsemen of the Apocalypse*, the fourth, or pale, horseman is variously described either as "death" or "pestilence."

Like many of the terms in this book, "plague" has a figurative dimension and is often used as a verb, for example, "Drug crime plagues the city." And we speak about mouse or rat plagues—think of the Pied Piper of Hamelin—and grasshopper plagues (though some prefer "grasshopper epidemics"), such as the locusts described in the Bible in the book of Exodus. The pied piper story concerns the death of just about all Hamelin's children. One speculation is that they were lured away to the disastrous (and perhaps equally mythical) Children's Crusade of 1212, while another idea is that their disappearance is a metaphor for what happened during a plague outbreak.

Do all pandemics involve infection?

One difficulty in all this is what we mean by "infection." The WHO definition strictly links pandemics to diseases caused by viruses, bacteria, and the like but, of late, this term is also being used to describe global trends for the increased incidence of chronic human conditions. Hence there is the Alzheimer's disease pandemic, the diabetes pandemic, the chronic obstructive pulmonary disease (COPD) pandemic, the cardiovascular disease pandemic, the obesity pandemic, and so on. There is plenty of medical evidence that viral and bacterial infections can play a part in the development of COPD, and may also be responsible for the early tissue damage that ultimately leads to some forms of diabetes and heart disease. However, it has not been possible to establish the sort of firm links that make a case for preventing diabetes or heart problems by, say, developing a vaccine against a particular pathogen.

Also, when we discuss obesity, cardiovascular disease, and diabetes, for example, what immediately comes to the fore is the cultural, profit-driven "pandemic" of "fast foods," carbonated drinks with high sugar content, and so forth that seems to be ever expanding in geographical reach. Morgan Spurlock's 2004 documentary *Supersize Me* tells how, if this type of diet doesn't kill you in the short term, it can definitely decrease your life expectancy. The U.S. government, for example, still spends billions of dollars in agricultural subsidies that both block export opportunities for poorer countries and support the production of extraordinarily damaging products like high fructose corn syrup. Europe is no better.

Then, there is the rapidly expanding cultural context that thrives on the contagion of random thoughts, attitudes, and information spread globally with incredible speed via web-based mechanisms like blogs, Twitter, Facebook, and YouTube. In the world of the Internet, "going viral" means that some story or idea has spread with incredible speed. Especially among the young, this more "democratic" web-based opinion is serving to dilute and even neutralize the misinformation and focus on the trivial that is the stock in trade of regressive newspaper editors, professional gossip columnists, radio "shock jocks," and so forth. At times, the Internet serves up examples of "good pandemics."

Describing the rapid dissemination of ideas and physiological conditions like obesity as a "pandemic" is undoubtedly legitimate by the criterion that many are affected and that the problem extends to more than two of the WHO regions. However, I will stick to the more traditional meaning: that of diseases caused by infectious microorganisms, particularly viruses. As discussed earlier, the viruses we're talking about here aren't patterns in cyberspace or code invented by some Internet saboteur but are physical entities that have some form of outer coat (protein, carbohydrate, and lipid), transmit their information via a nucleic acid (RNA or DNA) core, infect human beings (and other vertebrates), and primarily cause physiological problems.

What does the term "zoonosis" mean?

A zoonosis is simply an infection that transmits from animals to people. Though, as discussed in detail throughout this book, occasional zoonotic spread is the ultimate cause of many human disease outbreaks and ultimately pandemics, medical practitioners watch for a whole spectrum of familiar zoonotic infections that never evolve to spread horizontally between people. A classical example is the chronic, febrile debilitating disease toxoplasmosis, an infection caused by the protozoan *Toxoplasma gondii* that we typically contract from domestic cats. Pregnant women need to be particularly careful and practice scrupulous hand and other hygiene when around cats, as *T.gondii* can transmit vertically across the placenta and is a possible cause of miscarriage. Then there's hydatid disease, in which we contract the larval form of the sheep tapeworm (*Echinococcus granulosis*) by inadvertently ingesting food (or soil for a small child) that has been contaminated with dog feces. Big, fluid-filled hydatid cysts can then form in sensitive organs subsequent to the larvae invading across the gut wall and disseminating throughout the body. Prior to the introduction of effective public health measures that prevent dogs from consuming sheep offal, the removal of these space-occupying hydatid cysts was a major reason for neurosurgery in, for example, northern Greece.

On the other hand, while viruses like the 1968 Hong Kong flu that likely came into the human population from pigs and ducks (see Figure I.1) make the transition from being zoonotic to pandemic infections, the idea that a patient has contracted the flu from a source other than an infected human will be the last thing in the mind of your local doctor. The exception would be if someone presents with a very severe respiratory infection in a Southeast Asian country where the H5N1 bird flu is still active in domestic chicken populations.

In the strict etymological sense, an "epizootic" or "panzootic" is the animal equivalent of a human pandemic or epidemic. Tellingly, the terms "panzootic" and "epizootic" are now more commonly used by medical public health professionals than by those concerned with veterinary problems. During the course of a recent visit to Rome as part of the celebration and formal recognition of the global eradication of the cattle disease rinderpest, I realized that those associated with the UN Food and Agriculture Organization and the OIE (Organization Internationale des Epizootiques) prefer to use the terms "pandemic" and "epidemic" when describing the distribution profiles for veterinary infectious diseases. My personal view is that the terms "panzootic" and "epizootic" are redundant and, following current English usage, we might well consign them to the deep history of the language. "Pandemic" and "epidemic" should be sufficient for our purpose.

What is an endemic infection, and how does it differ from an epidemic infection?

Again, word usage is not all that precise. An *endemic infection* is one that has been well established over time in a particular institution, place, or demographic, whether local or worldwide. Diseases like HIV/AIDS and hepatitis C are endemic infections, though many would also think of them as the cause of continuing epidemics and pandemics. The dengue viruses, for example, which cause infections of limited duration, are maintained in a human/mosquito transmission cycle that is endemic to tropical regions such as Southeast Asia and the Caribbean. Such viruses spread north and south from their normal host range only when warm conditions are accompanied by heavy rainfall. Organisms like the typhoid- and cholera-causing bacteria are endemic to regions and populations in which there is no steady supply of clean water.

The term "endemic" can also be used in regard to potential pathogens that are ubiquitous in the environment but only become prominent when, for example, there is the possibility of widespread physical trauma as a consequence of violent conflict. Triggered by consistent dampness and unsanitary conditions, the fungal infection that caused trench foot was endemic to the northern European battlefields of World War 1. Further exposure of the damaged tissue to the ubiquitous soil bacterium *Clostridium perfringens* commonly led to gas gangrene, leaving surgeons with no alternative but to amputate. Regular changes of socks, together with rubbing whale fat into the feet, greatly reduced the incidence of this infectious disease. Gas gangrene, in which the anerobic (does not require oxygen) C. *perfringens* makes gas-producing toxins deep in muscle tissues subsequent to soil contamination of a gunshot, or other penetrating injury, continues to be a major problem where wounded combatants cannot get rapid access to medical or surgical intervention.

Are plants also included in the world of pandemics?

Following the epizootic/panzootic line for animals, the correct word for widely disseminated novel plant infections would probably be "epiphytic/panphytic," following the Greek *phytos* for plants. But an epiphytic (Greek *epi* for "upon" or "on") plant is one that parasitizes the surface of another, not something that spreads wildly across the environment. In fact, we talk about the pandemic of Dutch Elm disease caused by the fungus *Opheostoma ulmi*. It makes sense to set aside the fine points of philology and describe a widespread infection in any species as epidemic or pandemic.

In Summary

As is commonly the case, while terms like "pandemic," "epidemic," "outbreak," and "endemic" can be assigned precise meanings, as in the WHO pandemic influenza alert phases, they are also used in much less precise and overlapping ways. When you encounter evocative terms like "pandemic" and "epidemic" in dramatized personal accounts and, more generally, in the visual and print media, it's worth having a level of understanding that allows some critical assessment of how dangerous a developing situation may actually be.

3

THE SARS WARNING

Why was SARS so scary?

The problem with the 2002 outbreak of the severe acute respiratory syndrome, or SARS, was that it hit suddenly and people were dying horribly while both the cause and the principal mode of spread were unknown. Then, the epidemiology of SARS was very atypical for a respiratory pathogen. While the families of those who contract influenza are almost invariably and rapidly infected early on, that wasn't always the case with SARS. In fact, it didn't appear to transmit all that easily, though there was at least one situation in which the causative virus is known to have spread through an entire apartment building. Infected aerosols were apparently disseminated via dried-out U traps in floor drains, part of a poorly designed wastewater disposal system.

Another reason for the initial panic was that, unlike the situation for influenza, hospital personnel and other patients were at substantial risk of contracting SARS. As with influenza, the elderly were particularly susceptible, with about half of those aged 65 or older succumbing to the infection. Again, that's much worse than the normal situation for influenza, probably because there is some residual cross-reactive immunity from previous flu episodes experienced through a long lifetime. In the end analysis, though, SARS wasn't all that bad.

The SARS epidemic/pandemic started in November 2002 and was essentially over by July 2003. In all, there were only 9,000 confirmed cases, with less than 1,000 deaths. Contrast that with the recurring outbreaks of seasonal—normally cold weather—influenza that kill some 250,000–500,000 people globally each year, with about 10% of those being in the United States. The difference between SARS and seasonal influenza is that we are accustomed to the latter, have long known the cause, and a vaccine is often available. If it isn't, we know how to make vaccines and, as the necessary regulatory approvals are already in place in most countries, a product that provides protection against a new flu virus variant can generally be rolled out reasonably rapidly.

How did SARS spread so quickly through hospitals?

Though SARS didn't start in Singapore and the first cases outside mainland China were in Hong Kong, the story of the Singapore outbreak illustrates just how a hitherto unknown pathogen can, for a time, slip by even well-organized and perceptive medical scrutiny. The initial focus of infection in Singapore was the big Tang Tock Seng Public Hospital (TTSH). The "index" case, a 22-year-old, visited Hong Kong on a shopping trip and is thought to have contracted the infection while staying at a hotel known to be a primary site for SARS dissemination. On returning home, she became ill and was hospitalized at TTSH, where, very sick and fighting for breath, she was ultimately admitted to the intensive care unit. In all, this innocent tourist is considered to have passed the disease on to 24 people, including 9 hospital care workers who, at this early stage of the disease outbreak, were not wearing protective masks. She survived, but her mother, father, and another visitor all died.

That first patient also infected a 27-year-old nurse, who was later isolated, though not before she passed the disease on to 23 contacts. Those infected included a 53-year-old with diabetes and ischemic heart disease, who, because she had a number of medical problems and was not immediately identified as a SARS case, was transferred to the coronary care unit with severe congestive heart failure. She died after transmitting the disease to 25 more people. The diagnosis was also missed for a 60-year-old with chronic kidney disease and diabetes. Admitted to TTSH and discharged, he was then hospitalized again in an open ward at another hospital, Singapore General. There he started an outbreak involving 60 further cases. His brother visited and is thought to have transmitted the disease to 15 more people subsequent to being admitted to the National University Hospital.

Singapore has a sophisticated medical system with well-educated doctors and nurses, but, like most hospital professionals everywhere, hospital staff are overworked, often tired, and never have enough time. What this early Singapore experience illustrates is that in the absence of a specific, readily available laboratory test and a very high level of awareness, the variability of clinical presentation and the difficulty of differential diagnosis can lead to bad consequences. Modern medicine is effective only because of the underlying science and the resultant technology that facilitates the clear identification of the problem. Even then, it can take time to connect the dots.

The Singapore SARS story also provides a dramatic and extremely well-documented illustration of "nosocomial" spread. Nosocomial means simply that the infection is contracted in a health care facility. This is a well-recognized problem for multi-drug-resistant bacteria but, in the case of SARS, the spread within hospitals resulted simply from acuteness and novelty. The basic problem was that the pathogenesis of the infection, particularly the timing of maximum virus production and release, was simply not understood. All five Singapore SARS superspreaders (see below) were diagnosed in March, prior to the laboratory identification of the virus and the availability of diagnostic tests for patient monitoring.

What caused SARS and where did the pathogen come from?

Following a concentrated, collaborative effort by virus researchers in many centers, particularly Hong Kong, Paris, Vancouver, Atlanta, and Rotterdam, the cause of SARS was definitively established by April 2003, less than 6 months after clinicians and public health authorities first became aware of the disease. In April, the WHO announced that, working with a biotechnology company, the Bernard Nocht Institute in Hamburg had developed a PCR-based diagnostic kit, which was being made available at no cost to laboratories in the WHO collaborating network. Others established tests to detect SARS-specific antibodies in serum, the sure sign that an individual has been infected.

The SARS pathogen was new to science, though it does come from a well-known group (the coronaviruses, CoVs) that is commonly associated with mild sneezes, coughs, and colds in mammals. One CoV, infectious bronchitis virus, is a problem for meat and egg production in commercial chicken operations. Another has been implicated, along with many other viruses, as a possible cause of human multiple sclerosis (MS). But there is no proof that this is the case, though a related mouse virus, mouse hepatitis virus, is used as an experimental animal model of MS.

The initial conclusion was that the SARSCoV that caused the 2002–2003 outbreak had crossed over into the human population from Himalayan (or masked palm) civet cats (*Parguma larvata*). Civet cats bear no resemblance to our domestic *Felis catus* and indeed aren't even members of the felid family, which includes lions, tigers, panthers, cheetahs, and so on, all of which are carnivores. The masked palm civet cat, on the other hand, is a solitary, nocturnal, omnivore that eats anything (fruit or meat) that happens to be available. Civet cats are arboreal creatures that live in the forests of India and South Asia. How then did they come into contact with humans to transmit this infection? The answer is that, in parts of Asia, where many exotic species are used for human food, these little animals are hunted for sale and consumption, usually in restaurants. The SARS outbreak is thought to have originated from such a live animal market in the southern Chinese city of Guandong.

Sampling captive civet cats led to further SARSCoV isolations, while screening serum from animal handlers showed that many had antibodies to the virus, indicating that human infections may have been fairly common over the preceding years. This either went unrecognized or was not sufficiently serious to cause the local medical authorities to become involved. Particularly in areas where there are a lot of mosquitoes, non-specific fevers are fairly common, creating problems for differential diagnosis and obscuring novel infection events. What likely happened in late 2002 is that someone handling civet cats became infected with the SARSCoV and passed the disease on to others.

The mass movement across China that occurs during the Chinese New Year—when families travel to meet up, and when many festivals take place—may then have helped to spread the virus more widely. What is thought to have been critical is that some people are SARS "superspreaders" who, for reasons that are still not completely clear, excrete very large amounts of the virus into the external environment. One such superspreader brought the virus to Hong Kong, and separate individuals flew from there to Singapore and to Toronto, the only city that was affected outside the Asia/Pacific region.

The SARS outbreak is thus a classic example of what can happen when a novel pathogen first jumps across a species barrier to become established in a new host. And the molecular evidence continues to support the initial conclusion that the virus transferred from civet cats to humans, not the other way around. The SARSCoV that circulated in people has a deletion: that is, it has lost some of the genetic material found in the animal isolates.

A great deal of chance and randomness characterizes such crossover events. In the case of SARS, circumstances happened to come together—eating habits, timing, human movement patterns—in a way that resulted in a major problem. By the time the pandemic burned out, cases of SARS had been reported in 34 countries. Many of those who were clinically affected contracted the infection while traveling, and while some were sick enough to be hospitalized, most did not pass the disease on to cause local, secondary spread after returning home.

Aside from "natural" reservoirs, are there other potential sources of SARS?

After the outbreak was over, further research showed that the SARS virus is, in fact, endemic to bats, who would have in turn passed it to civet cats and, ultimately, to humans. As of March 2013, there have been 26 cases of severe respiratory disease in the Middle East, including 11 fatalities, that are known to have been caused by a related bat coronavirus. And there are four documented cases of scientists contracting SARS as a consequence of laboratory accidents since July 2003 with, in one instance, the infection spreading to 9 contacts, one of whom died. Subsequent investigation showed that the laboratories concerned were operating below standard and, since then, an Asian Pacific Biosafety Association (APBSA) has been established to train and monitor biosafety specialists. Some pathogens, including a few bacterial species (particularly the *Rickettsiae*), hepatitis B virus, and lymphocytic choriomeningitis virus, are notorious for infecting those who work in research and diagnostic laboratories. Much of this is historical, as biosafety equipment, security measures, and training procedures have been vastly improved over the past decades.

What steps were taken to stop the SARS outbreak?

The focus was always on limiting transmission, an effort that was greatly facilitated by the isolation of the virus and the development of convenient diagnostics. Early on, the Chinese authorities took just one week to build a tented isolation hospital in Beijing. Traveling at that time, I changed planes at Singapore airport to find that many on the concourse were wearing facemasks, which pretty much became a de rigueur dress accessory in SARS-afflicted cities. As arriving passengers walked toward the airport customs/immigration area, everyone's body temperature was taken by a remote sensor.

Once the pathogen was identified, it was an easy matter to work out where and when the virus was being excreted from patients, to keep such people in isolation, and to practice what is called "barrier nursing" while they were infectious. Antibody assays were soon developed to screen rapidly for evidence of recent or past exposure. Some simple experiments showed how well this virus survives outside the body.

What medical researchers soon realized is that, unlike influenza outbreaks, in which people are very infectious early on, the course of SARS is far more protracted. Again, the likely route of exposure with SARS is via the respiratory tract, where the virus first multiplies. However, unlike the situation for most respiratory pathogens (including influenza), the SARSCoV then infects white blood cells, which carry the virus around the body. That results in foci of virus growth in other tissues, including the gut mucosae, which in turn means that lots of virus can be present in stools. This more prolonged pathogenesis means that, again unlike influenza, where the virus infection may be well on the way to being controlled by the immune response before people are feeling really ill, those who were severely affected with SARS were still putting out a lot of virus at the time they were hospitalized. The net result was that doctors and nurses were particularly at risk, and a number of medical personnel died.

A further problem was that the SARSCoV is very resilient and survives well on hard surfaces (those aforementioned fomites) and in water. Hotel cleaners were programmed to wipe down elevator buttons at two-hour intervals. Grasping a stair rail or door handle that was contaminated as long as 24–48 hours previously could lead to infection if someone then picked his nose. The containment of SARs was thus achieved by quarantining severely affected individuals and by requiring those medical personnel who were in contact with them to wear gloves, gowns, and appropriate masks. Combining that with rigorous sanitation, especially hand-sterilization, and some (generally voluntary) restriction of movement brought the outbreak under control.

At this stage, there is no evidence that the SARSCoV is indeed circulating in humans. The threat is still out there, but should SARS return in any substantial way, we would know the nature of the problem within hours or days rather than months, as was the case in 2003. The exception would be, of course, an occurrence in an isolated community that "burns out" without coming to broader attention.

Did the SARS experience have long-term effects, and what lessons were learned?

SARS greatly increased international awareness of the danger that respiratory virus infections pose as a potential cause of pandemics, and it caused many countries, particularly China, to put more effort into "notifiable disease" surveillance mechanisms. As will be discussed in greater detail later, it took the Singapore economy about two years to recover from the effects of SARS, and the same was true of Hong Kong and Toronto. Recognizing the problem as early as April 2003, the Singapore government supplied a bailout of over $230 million. A retrospective analysis in 2005 concluded that SARS had cost Singapore $8 billion. That seems a pretty good reason for maintaining both a high level of infectious disease research and first-class public health facilities.

The medical effects of SARS were easier to absorb. Many of those who died were old and already clinically compromised as a consequence of various chronic disease problems. In the end, out of a total of 238 known cases, 33 people died from SARS in Singapore. Contrast that with the 193 road deaths there in both 2009 and 2010. But traffic accidents are just part of the normal "background" statistics, while a novel, rapidly spreading infection represents something entirely different. Schools were closed, and the direct financial effects on tourism, the airlines, the hotels, and business activity were both substantial and felt in the long term.

The essential point about SARS is that, while it was lethal for the elderly, many young people were much less severely affected. Combined with the fact that maximal levels of virus excretion were seen late, the movement of younger travelers provides a ready mechanism for disseminating the disease. Whether the SARS event should be called a pandemic is a moot point, though it is undoubtedly the case that, without the development of rapid containment mechanisms based on understanding the nature of this infection, SARS would have been much more widely disseminated around the globe. If the SARS incursion had, for example, occurred in the pre-tissue-culture days of the early twentieth century, it could well have taken off to be a global pandemic.

Also, though an example of international science detective work at its best, the identification of the SARS virus did not depend on novel insights or on the development of any new "platform" technology. Everything necessary for identifying this pathogen was already in place, including a combination of established international networks, the open exchange of material and reagents, the systematic and sensible application of state of the art science, and the availability of a vibrant biotechnology industry for the large-scale, rapid production of reliable reagents. Once researchers and clinicians had access to the PCR-based diagnostic kit for detecting the SARSCoV and antibody tests to check for evidence of infection, the SARS pandemic was consigned to history where, hopefully, it shall remain.

In a world where money and economics dominates international relations, SARS should teach us that no investment is more important than maintaining effective public health and disease surveillance mechanisms. With SARS, science protected humanity. We can only hope that this continues. Such protection comes at a financial cost: politicians and influential bureaucrats need to be kept in the loop so that the necessary resources continue to be provided.

4

TUBERCULOSIS AND INFLUENZA

Why should TB and influenza be considered together?

Apart from being respiratory pathogens, what links tuberculosis (TB) and flu is that they are old, very dangerous infections that simply will not go away. While SARS was an arriviste virus that flamed brightly and then faded back into obscurity, all those who monitor global infectious disease keep a very close watch on these traditional and too-familiar enemies.

What is the current situation with TB?

When it comes to bacterial infections, TB continues to be the respiratory disease that most concerns the WHO from the aspect of initiating a global pandemic. Caused by *Mycobacterium tuberculosis*, the TB bug probably came across into the human population from cattle sometime after the beginnings of agriculture about 10,000 years back, and it has been recognized as a major problem under various names (phthisis, consumption, the white plague) since the time of the Greeks. The cattle disease caused by the closely related *M. bovis* is now substantially controlled in most developed countries, with the main reservoirs of infection being in some wildlife populations, such as badgers in the United Kingdom. But *M. bovis* still infects humans from time to time and, historically, it's one of the reasons for pasteurizing milk. Heating milk briefly to at least 72 degrees Celsius (162°F) kills it off.

Beginning in the seventeenth century, Europe suffered a major TB epidemic with death rates among those infected through the 1800s as high as 25%. Many died young, including the poet John Keats and the composer Frederic Chopin. Somewhat simplistically, the TB bacteria invade lung macrophages, where they survive and provoke an ongoing inflammatory response, with invading (from the blood) T cells, B cells, and other macrophages cumulating to cause lumps, or granulomas, in the fragile respiratory tissue. These granulomas can erode small and even major blood vessels, with the result that patients cough up blood, a sign that death may be approaching from compromised lung function.

The virulent TB organism was first cultured by Robert Koch in 1882, and an attenuated (weakened) vaccine strain, BCG (Bacillus Calmette/Guerin), has been around for 90 years. While BCG can confer a measure of protection in some groups, the effect is variable, and it was never incorporated into the broader vaccination strategy of many countries, including the United States. Vaccinated infants are much less likely to develop tuberculous meningitis (infection of the brain), so BCG may be given to young children who are likely to be exposed. But, being a live bacterium, it cannot be used in any country where there is a high incidence of immunosuppression due to HIV/AIDS.

The retreat of "normal" TB as a cause of widespread mortality in the developed world reflects that the infection can be cured with antibiotics. However, because the bacteria tend to become anatomically "sequestered" and relatively inaccessible in lung granulomas, the therapy may need to be continued over a matter of months. Compliance can be a problem when the patient is psychologically dysfunctional, a situation seen commonly in intravenous drug users living on the streets. As a consequence, some jurisdictions have regulations that allow such people to be confined for "direct observed treatment" (DOT), over a time span that is being somewhat shortened with the development of better antibiotics. The epidemiologists calculate that a single infected individual has the potential to pass TB on to 12–15 others during a one-year period, so contact tracing by public health professionals is an obvious priority.

Before the development of the synthetic sulphaguanidines (sulfonamides, sulfa drugs) in the 1930s, and antibiotics in the mid 1940s, deprivation of liberty was also practiced for another bacterial disease, typhoid. Some will know the sad story of the Irish cook Mary Mallon, otherwise known as Typhoid Mary, a persistently infected carrier who spent almost 30 years of her life in enforced isolation after she infected a number of families in the New York City area. When Mary died, her gallbladder (which excretes its contents via the bile duct into the gut) was found to contain live *Salmonella typhi* bacteria. Apart from this disease being a continuing threat in developing countries, multi-drug-resistant (MDR) typhoid is an increasing problem.

Is multi-drug-resistant TB still an issue?

Very much so, and the TB story is far from unique, of course. The emergence of MDR bacteria (staphylococci, streptococci, and so forth) that cause distressing conditions like necrotizing fasciolitis (the so-called "flesh-eating bacteria") is being exacerbated globally by the "across the counter" sale and use of antibiotics, particularly in the developing world. There are also concerns about the practice of feeding antibiotics to (especially) pigs in the more prosperous countries. Such MDR bacteria are unlikely to cause pandemics, though they can be a major problem in hospitals. When it comes to MDR TB, the sense that the disease will remain a local problem is much less robust.

Until the early 1970s, infectious-disease specialists in the developed countries were still very wary of TB, but they also thought they had the measure of this terrible pathogen. That changed as a consequence of the 1982 emergence of the acquired immune deficiency syndrome, AIDS. The immune system collapse that, with time, develops in untreated HIV-infected individuals makes them very susceptible to severe infections caused by other organisms, with TB being prominent in that mix. Lack of any effective immune control means that AIDS patients replicate TB to a high level, a situation that favors the emergence of drug-resistant mutants. That effect, together with the lack of compliance mentioned earlier, is contributing to a higher international incidence of multi-drug-resistant TB, both in those with AIDS and throughout the broader community.

Apart from TB itself and the bovine variety, immunologically compromised AIDS patients can also be infected with *M. avium*—bird TB—and other "atypical" *mycobacteria*. Such "secondary," or "opportunistic," infections became much less of a problem with the development of anti-HIV "cocktails"— mixtures of various drugs—that stop the virus from destroying the immune system and prevent the development of AIDS. But by then, MDR TB had already emerged. And, of course, many in the developing world are either receiving no anti-HIV therapy, or are not being treated with the optimal cocktail of three antiviral drugs with differing modes of action. In general, those who are HIV positive are twice as likely to be infected with MDR TB.

People who live in Africa, parts of South America, and the Western Pacific countries may also be familiar with Buruli (Bairnsdale, Kumusi) ulcer, a slow developing skin infection caused by *M. ulcerans* that sometimes develops into a more generalized disease. Concurrent AIDS is a risk factor but, even in otherwise healthy individuals, large skin ulcers may need to be excised surgically, and the antibiotic treatment regime extends over at least 8 weeks. Skin trauma and biting insects are thought to be involved in transmission, and the infection is endemic in some Australian marsupials. This is another disease that is becoming more prevalent with the increased clearance or destruction of wetlands and forest habitats, though it is in no sense a pandemic threat.

What is being done to combat the MDR TB threat?

The threat from MDR TB is being monitored closely, though I should also tell you that the situation is in some ways worse than you think. The UN program that monitors AIDS globally (UNAIDS) is now recognizing an even more frightening phenomenon: the emergence of extreme drug-resistant (XDR) TB. Such variants are refractory to treatment with all known antibiotics and even the possibility of cure requires the administration of much rarer, more expensive, and often experimental drugs that have to be taken for up to 2 years. According to UNAIDS, XDR TB has now been reported from 45 countries, and we're also seeing TDR (total drug resistant) strains.

Clearly, given the high TB infection rates that prevailed in the days before antibiotics became available, the current situation is dangerous. However, organizations like the Bill and Melinda Gates Foundation and the Stop TB Partnership have been funding the development of novel anti-TB therapeutics. Recent estimates suggest that we should have new and effective drugs by the end of this decade, if not sooner. When it comes to antibiotics, what's been done so far has tapped relatively few of the possible biochemical pathways that could be exploited to kill an organism like *M. tuberculosis*. My personal view is that we should be optimistic and that, although TB should be closely monitored, the main danger when it comes to known respiratory infections continues to be the influenza A viruses.

Why might influenza remain the most obvious known pandemic threat?

There are a number of reasons. The first is that, of all the recurrent human respiratory virus infections, influenza causes the worst symptoms in substantial numbers of people, of all ages, everywhere. Lethal influenza pneumonia tends to be most common in the elderly, presumably because of the progressive (but variable) failure in immune function that accompanies aging. Still, though the available vaccines aren't always as effective as they might be in the elderly, it's worth hedging our bets by getting the shots. I'm now in my seventies and, working between the United States and Australia, often end up being "stuck" with both the Northern and Southern Hemisphere vaccine "cocktails" (which can vary) in the same year. Repeat vaccination boosts any existing level of immunity.

It is also the case that novel influenza "A" viruses, such as the one that caused the 1918–1919 pandemic and the 2009 swine flu, can sometimes cause a higher incidence of severe, acute respiratory failure in otherwise healthy young adults. That generally falls off in subsequent flu years when mutated, "seasonal" variants of the same virus strain are the continuing problem.

The second reason that influenza remains so dangerous is that these viruses grow very fast in the human respiratory tract, which means that people cough and sneeze aerosols containing virus particles even before they feel ill. Classically, other family members are infected early and, as people continue going to school or to their workplace, influenza spreads rapidly. Those who have a planned vacation or business trip think that the early signs of fever will soon pass, continue with their travel plans, and catch their flight.

Planes are the perfect transmitters, though not principally via the air that circulates generally through the cabin. Even so, the epidemiological evidence suggests that there is a risk of contracting the infection from people sitting up to two rows away from you. A fifteen-minute conversation with a fellow passenger increases the likelihood of droplet transmission, and being in an aisle seat may also add a marginal element of danger. Mostly though, planes just spread influenza by moving infected people quickly to new places. There is well-documented evidence that a "seasonal" influenza virus can spread across the United States in 6 weeks and around the world in less than 6 months.

A further reason is that the influenza A viruses, at least, are constantly changing. As a consequence, a vaccine that protects people one year may be less effective or even useless the next. This means that new vaccines need to be made and distributed annually or even bi-annually with, as mentioned above, different variants being used for protection in the Northern and Southern Hemispheres. That need for constant revision and revaccination may provide some benefit for the companies producing these products, but it is an expensive and cumbersome way of doing things. Also, it can take months to adapt a newly isolated influenza virus, then produce and distribute the vaccine for it, and the WHO committee that makes these decisions has to decide some 8 months ahead of time what viruses are likely to be circulating in different regions during the coming influenza season. All prediction is probabilistic. There's always a chance of making the wrong decision. And that has happened with influenza.

What are the different kinds of influenza viruses?

So far I've mostly talked about the influenza A viruses, but there are also B and C viruses. The A and B lists concern us most. Influenza C virus causes occasional outbreaks in humans and pigs, though the symptoms are usually mild. The disease profiles for the influenza A and B viruses are essentially identical. The standard so-called triple influenza vaccine normally contains two influenza A viruses and an influenza B virus. Both types can change, however, by the process that researchers call "antigenic drift." "Antigen" refers to the components (generally proteins) on the surface of the virus (see Figure 1.2 in Chapter 1) that are recognized by the body's protective antibodies (Ig), while "drift" refers to the process of mutational change in the viral RNA that leads in turn to alterations in protein structure and "escape" from Ig binding.

These spontaneous events are not necessarily dangerous, as any mutation can have a "fitness cost" that compromises the capacity of the virus to reproduce itself. To expand on this idea, the survival of influenza viruses depends ultimately on their capacity for transmission. If the original, or wild type, influenza virus (X) that's replicating in the respiratory tract cells of an infected person still grows faster than the mutant (Y) that emerges in the lung of the same individual, then it's much more likely that X will be transmitted to someone else, with the consequence that the Y mutant will be a "dead end" that goes nowhere.

The mutations that concern us most are in the genes that encode the hemagglutinin (H) and neuraminidase (N) proteins located on the outside of the virus particle (see Figure 1.2 in Chapter 1). The function of the H molecule is to bind ubiqui tous sialic acid (carbohydrate) molecules on the cell surface, an event that triggers the necessary process of virus interiorization into the cytoplasm. The N does precisely the opposite job, acting as an enzyme to cleave and break off the H-sialic acid interaction and allow the escape of newly made progeny virus from the cell. The anti-influenza drugs *Tamiflu* (oseltamivir) and *Relenza* (zanamivir) function by binding to the active site on the N molecule in a way that blocks this cleavage/release mechanism. As a consequence, the new virus particles "hang up" at the cell surface, and the spread of the infection through the respiratory tract is delayed until the slowly developing (5–7 days in the unvaccinated) adaptive immune response catches up and eliminates those virus-producing factories, the infected cells.

In a typical influenza infection, an incoming influenza virus particle from an aerosol or hand/nose contact can be "taken out" in a vaccinated person by preexisting antibodies that bind segments of the H or N glycoproteins. This prevents infection and "labels" the virus for consumption (phagocytosis) and destruction by the specialized macrophages (literally, "big eater" cells) that are distributed along much of the airway surface in the lungs. Influenza virus-strain-specific neutralizing antibodies circulate in the cell-free plasma fraction of the blood and "seep through" to the protective mucus layer. They can also be made at the infection site by the plasma cells, antibody-producing factories that have located to immune nodules in the lung, the bronchus-associated lymphoid tissue. These mechanisms are discussed in more detail in the first chapter.

What happens with the H protein molecule illustrates biological evolution at its simplest. As the population is progressively protected by specific immunity—perhaps generated during the process of recovery from a currently circulating influenza strain, perhaps by prior vaccination—the ideal situation develops for the selection of any variant virus with an escape (from neutralizing antibody binding) mutation in the H molecule. The net result is the antigenic drift that gives rise to the seasonal influenza A and B viruses that spread globally every year or two. We don't refer to such outbreaks as pandemics, even though, at least so far as the H antigen is concerned, the seasonal virus is essentially novel as it hasn't been seen before. Pandemic influenza is reserved for the case where a previously unencountered (by humans) influenza A virus emerges from nature as a consequence of antigenic shift. The influenza B viruses don't shift, so the variant B strains are essentially seasonal in character.

What is antigenic shift and why is it so dangerous?

The hereditary information of the influenza A viruses (see Figure 1.2 in Chapter 1) is organized into 8 discrete RNA segments (or genes). If a cell is infected simultaneously with two different strains, the 16 RNA sets derived from the two parents can re-package (or re-assort) to give a novel virus, again with the 8 complementary genes that allow virus replication. That experiment is readily done in the laboratory and also occurs from time to time in nature. The H3N2 Hong Kong flu of 1968 is an example of such an antigenic shift (see Figure I.1) and is thought to have emerged when a cell in the respiratory tract of a susceptible mammal, likely a human or a pig, was infected at the same time with the then-circulating "human" H2N2 "Asian flu" virus and an H3N8 "duck" virus. Avian and human influenza A viruses bind slightly different sialic acid receptors, with both being readily available in the pig lung. That makes the pig an ideal "mixing vessel." Humans can catch influenza from pigs, and the reverse is also true.

The influenza A viruses are generally ubiquitous among water birds (see Figure 4.1), with there being 16 different known H and 9 N types. Replicating in cells of the GI (rather

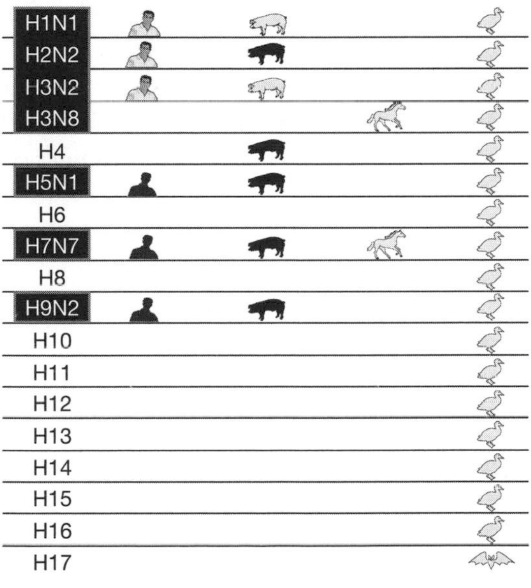

Figure 4.1. Aquatic birds are known to be the reservoir hosts for influenza A viruses with 16 different H and 9 different N types. In addition, the isolation of a novel "H17" influenza virus from South American fruit bats was reported in early 2012. As can be seen, the flu strains that have become established in us are all of the H1N1, H2N2 or H3N2 "serotypes." Humans are occasionally infected with H5N1, H7N7, H7N9 and H9N2 viruses and, apart from H5N1 and the possible return of H2N2, viral epidemiologists are concerned that an H9N2 virus could possibly jump to us. As to viruses of the less-common H types, it may just be random chance that has kept these strains out of human populations.

Reproduced courtesy of Dr. Robert G. Webster at St. Jude Children's Research Hospital.

than respiratory) tract, virus particles are voided from the bird's cloaca, the common orifice of the avian GI and urogenital tracts. The fact that the influenza A viruses survive well in water then ensures that, as different bird populations come together on inland lakes and waterways, a variety of species will be infected. That provides an ideal mechanism for distributing a dangerous pathogen. The hi-path H5N1 variant that emerged in 2005 to kill geese and swans on Quinghai Lake in western China was far less virulent for ducks, which spread the infection westward to India, the Middle East, Europe, and North Africa. Most of these avian H and N types aren't a problem for humans. The four human influenza pandemics of the past century were caused by a very limited spectrum (H1N1, H2N2, or H3N2) of influenza A virus variants. Then there is the emerging situation in China where 126 people have developed severe clinical disease and 26 have died following infection with an avian H7N9 virus, though there is as yet no evidence of horizontal spread between humans. This is the first report of H7N9 infections in humans.

But birds aren't the only source of pandemic influenza A viruses, as the 2009 SW flu showed by its very name. What is believed to have happened here is that two "swine" H1N1 strains (imported Eurasian and local North American) swapped some genes following a chance, simultaneous infection of a Mexican pig (Figure 4.2). This led to the emergence of a novel, "reassorted" H1N1 virus that proved highly infectious for humans. This strain displaced the current "seasonal" H1N1 influenza A virus, "drifted" variants of which had been circulating in people for years. Both the SW H1 and the internal nucleoprotein genes of the 2009 human pandemic strain were, in fact, very similar to those of the 1918 H1N1 pandemic virus. Way back in 1918, the virus that killed so many people also became established in pigs where, though it ultimately burned out and disappeared from the human population, it remained relatively unchanged over the years.

Recently, these pig viruses have been reassorting at a much higher rate than seen hitherto. From July 2011 to December

H1N1 Pandemic Influenza – 2009
Source of Gene Segments

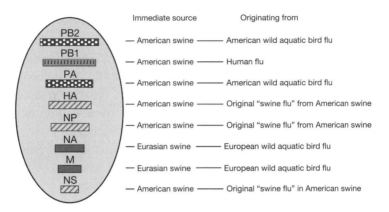

Figure 4.2. This figure illustrates the likely origin of the different flu genes that reassorted from viruses circulating separately in Eurasian and North American pigs to give a novel pathogen that was highly infectious for us. How the "Eurasian" virus got to Mexico is not known. The mixing event could have happened somewhere else, with the new pandemic virus coming to Mexico in the lung of an infected human traveler. The swine H1N1 viruses are considered to be fourth-generation descendants of the 1918 human pandemic strain. These viruses changed less in pigs than in us. The NP gene, for example, is very similar to that found by Taubenberger and colleagues when they "resurrected" the 1918 pathogen. It should be emphasized that, while an initial virus crossover must reflect that at least one person became directly infected with a virus from a pig, we normally catch the flu from people, not pigs (or birds). It's safe to eat cooked pork, chicken, or duck.

Reproduced courtesy of Dr. Robert G. Webster at St. Jude Children's Research Hospital.

2012, a pig virus identified as H3N2v is known to have infected 319 people in 11 U.S. states. All were in people who had significant contact with pigs at agricultural fairs, and there has been little evidence of community spread. Though this virus has not been particularly infectious, there seems a good possibility that the next human pandemic strain will again emerge from the swine reservoir. The concern is, of course, that this could reflect the mixing of a pig virus with one of the hi-path H5N1 avian strains that continue to circulate in parts of Asia.

Even if that mixing did occur, there is no certainty that the emergent virus would be nearly as lethal as the variants that continue to cause periodic mortality in bird populations and have (since 1997) also killed 60% of the 500-plus people who are known to have developed symptoms. The high mortality rate is thought to reflect that those who contracted the disease breathed a large dose of virus deep into their lungs where, unlike in the upper respiratory tract, both the avian and mammalian sialic acid receptor sites that bind the viral H molecule can be found together. So far, though there have been occasional hints that this might have occurred, there is little evidence that the H5N1 virus spreads between humans.

Are birds and pigs our main concern when it comes to catching the flu?

No, infected people are the big danger. When it comes to respiratory infections including influenza, babies and small children are infinitely more dangerous than birds or pigs, especially for fond grandparents with failing immune systems. Even so, well-documented cases of H3N2v infections in agriculture-oriented humans through 2011–2012 (see above) emphasize that it is possible to catch this disease from a pig. If your pet mini-pig starts to sneeze, put it in quarantine for a couple of weeks. The severe influenza season throughout the United States in late 2012, early 2013, was substantially due to s seasonal variant of the H3N2 virus that had long been circulating in humans, not the pig-origin H3N2v strain.

And the likelihood of contracting influenza from an infected bird is extremely small, even for those of us who live in regions where the high-path H5N1 virus remains active in chicken and water bird populations. It may not be a good idea to nuzzle up to a parrot, but if you do subsequently develop a fever and respiratory symptoms, tell your doctor. The probable diagnosis will be the bacterial infection psittacosis, a disease that is readily treated with antibiotics.

Other avian influenza strains occasionally cause problems in humans. Checking serum antibodies from those who work with poultry can give evidence of prior exposure to H7 and H9 avian influenza A viruses. In a 2003 H7N7 avian influenza outbreak that took place in the Netherlands, the vigorous efforts to cull and control the infection in domestic chickens led to 89 verified symptomatic cases in humans. It was very hot and, while those involved were provided with protective clothing, few used it properly. A veterinarian died, but most of those infected had mild upper respiratory tract infections and conjunctivitis. Interestingly, there was also evidence of person-to-person spread, though that was not appreciated clinically at the time and only came to light following subsequent antibody testing. In general and so far as that's possible, it's probably a good idea to maintain a reasonable distance from all "snotty nosed" (or runny-beaked) creatures.

What is most important is to maintain your influenza vaccination status. That should ensure that you do not become the mammalian mixing vessel (see Figures 1.2 and 4.1) in which a pig (or bird) virus and a currently circulating human strain get together to make a new, reassorted variant that goes on to cause a dangerous pandemic. If that happened in the United States, it's not unlikely that the CDC would track you down. Living or dead, you would be famous, but for the wrong reasons.

What was so special about the virus that caused the 1918–1919 influenza pandemic?

It is, as we've seen, the most deadly influenza pandemic of modern times, so of course we have to return to it again and again. What was special about it has only been understood recently. Back in 1918, though influenza was clearly infectious, those investigating the pandemic were unable to isolate and identify the causative agent. The first demonstration that influenza was caused by a virus came some 12 years later, in 1933, when Richard E. Shope of the Rockefeller Institute (now Rockefeller University) branch laboratory in Princeton, New Jersey, transmitted influenza between pigs, using fluid that had been passed through filters with pore sizes that would hold back the much larger bacteria and fungi.

That same year, Wilson Smith, the young Christopher Andrewes—of later Common Cold Unit fame—and colleagues working in the Medical Research Council Laboratories at Mill Hill, on the outskirts of London, caused pneumonia in ferrets by exposing them to throat garglings from Andrewes, who had a bad case of the flu. The ferrets further fulfilled Robert Koch's postulates for determining the cause of a transmissible disease by in turn giving the infection to Charles Stuart Harris, a junior researcher in the group.

By 1933, of course, at least with the technology available at that time, any possibility of recovering live influenza virus from those who had died over a decade earlier seemed long gone. Still, some degree of categorization was possible. Testing serum antibodies in survivors showed that the virus circulating back then could be classified as an H1N1 strain. That meant it was related to the 1933 isolate transmitted to ferrets by the Mill Hill scientists. Their H1N1 virus—officially called A/WSN/1933— is still used today in research laboratories. Like a few extremely virulent flu viruses (including H5N1), this virus can cause neuropathology in some laboratory animal species.

That is how things stood until the enormous technological surge forward in molecular science that resulted from the development of the PCR technique we discussed earlier. Working at the U.S. Armed Forces Institute of Pathology in Washington, D.C., in 1996, Jeffrey Taubenberger and his group—including Ann Reid and Amy Krafft—succeeded in expanding much of the virus genome from paraffin-embedded blocks (used for more than a century by pathologists to cut histological sections) of lung tissue taken from young soldiers who died acutely in 1918 army recruit camps. Then, in collaboration with Johan Hultin, who had been trying to recover live virus from people who had been buried quickly (and thus flash-frozen) in the Alaskan permafrost, the team was progressively able to reconstruct the entire 1918 H1N1 virus genome.

When given to non-human primates, laboratory mice, and ferrets under high-security conditions, this resurrected virus has proved as virulent as the hi-path H5N1 influenza strains.

A major furor erupted in late 2011 when it was reported that two leading influenza research groups had used serial passage to adapt the virulent, avian H5N1 virus for transmission between ferrets and (possibly) humans. This taught us two things that we needed to know: first, that these H5N1 viruses can potentially change in ways that may facilitate their transmission from person to person; second, it allowed the identification of specific mutations in the viral RNA that could then be monitored for emergence in naturally occurring "field" variants. An intense debate that played out in the popular media asked whether such studies should ever have been done and, if so, whether the results should be published openly for all to read, including possible terrorists. The scientists in the field declared a moratorium and shut down the research so that the issue could be thoroughly discussed in an appropriate forum. After some tightening of the criteria, the moratorium ended in early 2013, though the discussion is far from over. A very real danger is that someone who is under-qualified and working in a sub-standard laboratory environment could do such experiments. That's not likely to happen in any well-regulated medical research system, but the technologies are far from obscure and responsible countries like the United States can no longer hope to control what happens globally.

What have we learned so far concerning the origins of the 1918 virus? The gene sequence is broadly avian-like, but there does not seem to be a strong case for arguing that it came directly from some bird reservoir. Neither is there evidence that it emerged as a consequence of a mixing event (reassortment) in a pig. The progenitor remains unknown. Taubenberger is interested in going back to do the "molecular archaeology" of viruses that were circulating in people prior to 1918, but it is an extremely difficult task, as the likelihood of finding suitable, well-identified post mortem material is low.

Is our capacity to counter influenza improving?

Knowledge is power, and we are certainly far better equipped to deal with a novel influenza A virus than we were in 1918, 1957, or 1968, when the pandemic flu viruses of the twentieth century emerged (see Figure I.1) That's true from a number of aspects, including public health policy and surveillance, vaccine availability, and preventive/therapeutic approaches, such as antibiotics to deal with secondary bacterial pneumonia and oxygen therapy. Also, there's a great deal of innovative research currently in process, and it's likely that we will see substantial improvements in making a lot of vaccine fast to prevent infection, and in treating those with severe symptoms, over the next decade or two.

Though the origin of the 1918 H1N1 virus remains obscure, the 1957 Asian (H2N2) and 1968 Hong Kong (H3N2) pandemic influenza A viruses are both thought to have emerged from "traditional" agricultural communities in which people, domestic birds, and pigs live close together under warm, humid conditions. Such conditions are prevalent in Southeast Asia. The end of wars—such as in Cambodia and Vietnam—and the increasing technical sophistication of many Pacific-rim nations, along with the need to counter the continuing (since 1997) avian H5N1 challenge, has led to influenza being a priority disease for both medical and veterinary surveillance.

In order to step up surveillance efforts, a WHO facility was built in Beijing in 2007, adding to the four other WHO Collaborating Centers for Influenza (London, Atlanta, Melbourne, Tokyo) and the one animal center (Memphis, Tennessee). Partially funded by the United States, a major program based in Hong Kong University is in the ideal location to monitor virus incursions from both the East and the West. Apart from the involvement of leading scientists, advances in the technology of DNA sequencing that go under names like "pyro sequencing" and "deep sequencing" allow the very rapid detection of novel mutations that could, for example, emerge as new seasonal flu strains. Once a given influenza

A virus is established and circulating in humans, the mutations that lead to the emergence of new seasonal variants can, of course, occur anywhere and at any time.

Beginning with the 2002–2003 SARS experience, then the H5N1 scare and the 2009 SW flu pandemic, a broadly increased consciousness of the medical and economic damage that can result from rapidly spreading diseases like influenza caused both governments and private enterprises to take virulent respiratory infections very seriously. National and local preparedness plans were either initiated or upgraded, increased resources were allocated to both basic and applied influenza research, and better surveillance mechanisms were put in place at airports. Whether the temperature detectors located in the immigration area at some international airports to monitor incoming passengers as they walk by are technically effective is a matter of debate, but they do help to increase awareness for both staff and travelers. Logically, in fact, it would be more sensible to screen people before they board the aircraft.

Are we making progress with flu vaccines?

There's a lot of research going on in this area, and both the quality and the quantity of the vaccines that are being made have been steadily improving. Nevertheless, the problem remains that, when a novel pandemic or seasonal strain emerges out of nowhere, it still takes about 6 months to get any vaccine out into the broader community. The reasons vary. One is that most influenza vaccines are still grown in embryonated hen's eggs. As a consequence, there aren't many places with the necessary equipment to produce the vaccine. Some influenza vaccine is now made in cell cultures, offering a greater spectrum of production facilities. However, cultured cells still tend to make less vaccine virus than chick embryos. The influenza A viruses are primarily avian in origin, so it's not surprising that they grow well in bird tissues.

The amount of virus (and thus virus protein) is a major issue when it comes to producing the standard, inactivated (killed), non-replicating influenza vaccines. One recent advance that may turn out to be very important (though, alas, it did not work well for the 2009 H1N1 pandemic strain) is the development and testing of a novel "reverse genetics" technology for producing influenza vaccines. Necessitated by the fact that the H5N1 viruses were rapidly proving lethal to chick embryos, the reverse genetics strategy allowed virologists to "engineer" the avian H5 and N1 genes into the other gene "backbone" of a standard laboratory influenza strain that grows well in eggs and/or cell cultures. That procedure can now be followed with any newly isolated influenza A virus.

And it now seems possible that the rapid production problem for flu vaccines may have been cracked using a very different approach. Very recent reports indicate that the viral H molecule can be produced rapidly and in large quantities using cultured cells from the ovary of the fall armyworm. So far, these are media stories in generally responsible formats, but we have yet to see the actual evidence published in the science literature.

Attenuated, live influenza virus vaccines that replicate only at the lower temperatures found in the human upper respiratory tract (nose and oropharynx) were long used in the former Soviet Union and are now available in the United States (*Flumist*). Though they are yet to be approved for the very young or the elderly, these vaccines do have the advantage that, because they multiply in the nose and upper respiratory tract of those given the product, it is not necessary to grow as much virus to put in the vaccine vials. However, the attenuated viruses—also known as "cold-adapted viruses"—suffer from the problem that besets all influenza vaccines: there is little time for extensive human safety testing in the face of a pandemic.

That created a problem with one of the standard "killed" vaccines in Australia recently, when a product made using well-established protocols proved to be more reactogenic than usual, causing unacceptable levels of high fever—and occasional convulsions—in a few young children. Given that a new vaccine is made to protect against a novel virus, even of a broadly familiar type, there can be no absolute guarantee against unpredicted side effects. Ultimately, the use of any such preventive is determined by a benefit/risk equation that will not be fully comprehended until thousands, or millions, have been exposed. If we look at the 2009 H1N1 SW pandemic there were, for example, more than 340 confirmed pediatric flu deaths in the United States.

No fatalities were definitively attributed to the administration of that "reactogenic" Australian vaccine, but there were some disturbing correlations, including an infant who died within 24 hours of being dosed. Febrile convulsions are mainly a problem for small children. What may be needed here is a bioassay that can be used to test serum from a few vaccinated adults to see if the product in question causes abnormal production of the molecules (cytokines/chemokines) that are known to cause fever. Such technology is readily available. But the idea would first have to be tested in adults and then, if found to be useful, made part of the regulatory requirement for licensing killed influenza vaccines.

Another area of research focuses on the development of new adjuvants, or substances that are added to a vaccine to increase the levels of antibody production. One commonly used product is the chemical compound alum; another is the oil-in-water preparation MF59, or squalene. Then there's a spectrum of naturally made biological products that are emerging as a consequence of the current focus on the character of innate immunity. Increasingly, we are coming to understand how molecular events that occur very early in the course of an infection function to promote the more specific, and later, adaptive immunity that gives long-term immune memory.

The "Holy Grail" with influenza would be to produce a universal vaccine, though many doubt that this is a realistic goal. The vaccine producers already have a profitable product that has to be given repeatedly, and there is a question of whether any government would be willing to find the $1 billion or more that would be required to see this through. Still, a great deal of current research focuses on the possibility that stimulating the more cross-reactive (between influenza A viruses) CD8+ T cell memory compartment could pave the way for a more rapid response—one that diminishes the severity rather than totally prevents the consequences of infection with a broad spectrum of influenza strains. Going for partial protection rather than sterilizing immunity has real advantages, since mild infections are likely to boost existing, cross-reactive immunity, which in turn keeps the levels of both T cell and B cell memory high and helps to minimize the severity of subsequent challenges with different influenza viruses.

Other cross-reactive vaccine strategies are directed at "tricking" the immune system by focusing the antibody response onto "shared" regions of the virus H molecule, or at targeting immunity to the conserved M2 ion channel protein that is found at low abundance (relative to H and N) on the surface of the influenza virus particle (Figure 1.2). My personal view is that the broad-spectrum influenza vaccine strategies currently under development have a long way to go. However, given the intensity of the focus on research into both influenza and HIV/AIDS, where the vaccine problem is in many respects similar, it is possible that there may be rapid advances. And, if we are able to develop such a universal influenza vaccine, the public health question would then be whether it should be used as a regular counter to seasonal influenza, or held in strategic reserve to counter a completely novel flu A strain. Another possibility would be to give it, say, every 3 years, to boost existing, cross-reactive immunity.

Apart from vaccines, are there other products available to prevent infection?

Earlier, I mentioned the neuraminidase blockers *Relenza* (zanamivir) and *Tamiflu* (oseltamivir), which can be used to protect key medical personnel and those who provide essential services, such as border protection and food delivery. These drugs, which block any influenza A or B virus, were purchased in bulk at the time of the H5N1 pandemic scare, and there is some evidence that, when given to those with early symptoms, they did help to blunt clinical severity in the initial phases of the 2009 H1N1 SW flu pandemic. The problem is that they are very expensive, limited in supply, and that the more they are given the more rapidly some drug-resistant virus will emerge. Resistance to *Tamiflu* (though not *Relenza*) is, for example, widespread for the H1N1 (but not the H3N2) influenza A viruses. Then there is the long-acting neuraminidase inhibitor *Inavir* (laninamivir), which has recently been licensed for human use in some countries. A single, inhaled dose of *Inavir*, for example, has been shown to protect influenza virus-challenged mice for at least a week. Other antivirals that target different molecular pathways required for influenza virus replication are also being developed.

Finally, as discussed briefly in the earlier chapter on infection and immunity, researchers have succeeded in isolating the relatively rare (occurring a frequency of less than one in a million) B lymphocytes/plasma cells that produce antibodies specific for cross-reactive regions (shared determinants) on the virus H molecule. Such human mAbs can, like the similar therapeutics available for the treatment of some tumors (*Herceptin* for breast cancer, *Ibrutomab* for non-Hodgkin's lymphoma), be produced in bulk using recombinant DNA technology. Compared with small molecule therapeutics (drugs), the mAbs have the advantage of a longer half-life ($t_{1/2}$), or persistence in blood. In general, mAb therapy is being rapidly advanced by molecular engineering approaches aimed at increasing the affinity (or tightness) of binding and the duration of plasma bio-availability. The downside to such research is expense and the fact that, if and when it does come to a respiratory infection pandemic, the product would have to be injected—meaning done by an MD or allied medical professional. In general, anything that brings people together in doctors' offices or emergency rooms during a pandemic is an obvious risk factor.

How afraid should we be of influenza?

Maintaining a good level—above inactivity, below panic—of awareness and, particularly if you are older, taking advantage of the opportunity for annual immunization against the seasonal influenza A and B viruses make sense. The statistics indicate that repeat flu vaccination is generally correlated with a reduced incidence of illness and hospitalization and greater longevity. Better immune protection is no doubt part of the reason, though this correlation between vaccine uptake and more robust health may also reflect that those who live well and are financially secure are more likely to see a doctor when any problem arises.

It is important to seek medical help if you do develop any severe respiratory disease. While the initial cause may be a virus that—beyond the earliest stage of infection when a drug like *Relenza* may be useful—is not susceptible to anything other than symptomatic treatment, primary (caused by *Streptococcus, Haemophilus, Mycoplasma, Chlamydia, Klebsiella*, or *Legionella* species) and secondary bacterial pneumonias can be treated with antibiotics. Producing snot and coughing up phlegm that is darker yellow to greenish in color is suggestive that bacteria may be involved, though that is by no means certain, and the final judgment needs to be made by an experienced medical practitioner.

When it comes to vaccines against endemic infections, it's also a good idea for older people (and children, of course) to be protected against the pneumococcal disease caused by *Streptococcus pneumoniae*. Another risk is from the ubiquitous respiratory syncytial virus (RSV), which is particularly dangerous for young babies and can kill residents of nursing homes. Vaccines are in development (though not currently available) and there is a virus-specific mAb (*Palivizumab)* that can be used to protect vulnerable infants. Though there are no vaccines, the coronaviruses and parainfluenza viruses that cause colds and croup in the young can also be much more problematic for the elderly.

The bottom line is that pulmonary infections are dangerous, especially for young infants (because they have very small airways) and for older people. Any severe—especially if accompanied by fever—or persistent respiratory symptoms should be checked by a well-qualified professional. You would be both unlikely and very unlucky to become infected with MDR or TDR tuberculosis, but it isn't impossible. When it comes to an epidemic or pandemic situation, listen to what the responsible authorities are saying and behave accordingly. That will be discussed in greater detail later. In the case of influenza, take the available vaccines ahead of time and see a doctor early if symptoms develop, particularly if the afflicted individual is in a high-risk category. The present flu vaccines do not provide 100% protection, especially in the elderly. As mentioned earlier, the 2012–2013 winter flu season was associated with widespread illness in the United States. Many who missed their shots made the effort once they realized there was a problem. That was certainly the case in Boston, perhaps the worst affected city in late 2012, where people formed long lines to get the influenza vaccine, which was then in short supply.

5

FLEDERMAUS TO FIELD MOUSE

What's a fledermaus?

Fledermaus is German for bat, literally, "a flying mouse." Bats are the most abundant mammals on earth. Fruit bats did get a mention with the SARS virus, of course, but there's a much bigger and scarier story to tell here. This chapter will also discuss the horrible pathogens carried by a number of small furry creatures, particularly various species of wild mice that live a very grounded lifestyle.

Is it unusual that fruit bats carry SARS?

No, although the still-emerging story that fruit and insect bats carry a whole range of viruses that can potentially infect us has been a big surprise for everyone. A decade back, the only situation we knew about where a virus passed commonly from bats to other warm-blooded mammals was for rabies transmitted to cattle—and occasionally humans—by hematophagous, or blood-sucking, vampire bats. Apart from accidental exposure to aerosols in a laboratory or the inadvertent transplant of corneas from an infected individual, rabies is generally contracted as a result of being bitten. That's because the virus is present at high concentration in the salivary glands. Dogs pose the greatest risk, though raccoons, foxes, and other wildlife are also dangerous. It is very important to avoid handling any sick wild animal, especially in countries where rabies is endemic.

The bat-rabies problem was essentially restricted to South America, where the vampires of the subfamily *Desmondontiae* are found, though there has long been speculation about the possibility that insectivorous and fructiverous (fruit-eating) bats may also carry and spread this virus. While such bat species don't normally attack humans and other mammals, they do have teeth and strong jaws for biting through the tough rinds of tropical fruits. Especially if sick and behaving abnormally as a consequence of the damage caused to the brain by a rabies-like virus, they can bite if handled. When bats invade a human living space, their removal should be left to professionals. Bats other than the vampire varieties are now known to carry related lyssaviruses. A licensed bat-handler in Scotland and two Australians have died as a consequence of such infections, one from an insectivorous bat. In Australia, where there is no evidence of rabies in dogs or wildlife, all bat handlers are now given the standard rabies vaccine. Is it just a matter of chance that these Australian lyssaviruses have not become established in domestic or wild dogs?

Rabies is a terrible disease, but it doesn't pose a grave pandemic threat. We have long had the tools, including good vaccines needed to deal with that infection. The first rabies vaccine was, in fact, developed in 1885 by Emil Roux and was used successfully by Louis Pasteur. And apart from vaccination, the extent of the rabies problem can be greatly mitigated by sound public health measures, like culling and sterilizing wild dogs while vaccinating domestic pets and at-risk livestock. Some countries, like Australia, have kept rabies out by quarantine. Where the virus is endemic, as in the United States, there is always the risk of encountering an infected fox, skunk, or raccoon. Both in Europe and North America, there has been some success in vaccinating wildlife by dropping baits, chicken heads laced with an "attenuated" rabies vaccine, from light planes.

Also, while rabies was once almost invariably fatal, being bitten by a rabid dog today is not necessarily a death sentence. Professional help should be sought as soon as possible and, even if there is a delay for some reason, it is still important to initiate treatment. As discovered many years ago by Pasteur and his colleagues, rabies is one of the few infections where post-exposure vaccination can prevent the development of disease. These bullet-shaped viruses travel slowly along the nerve fibers, so if the entry point is the foot, the leg, or even the hand, there can be enough time for an effective immune response to develop before the virus reaches the brain. But in the nerves, rabies remains "hidden" from the immune system, which is why it is necessary to give the vaccine.

Because the nerve tracts are so much shorter, the prognosis is much worse for someone bitten on the face, or for a laboratory worker who accidentally contracts the infection as a consequence of inhaling an aerosol containing rabies virus, perhaps released from a shattered test tube or following an accident associated with some brain tissue homogenization procedure. The virus can potentially go directly from the back of the nose, via the olfactory nerves to the olfactory (smell) centers of the brain. Also, several people have died as a consequence of being given corneal grafts from undiagnosed rabies cases. Recent developments in the area of mAb therapy may, however, provide some hope when it comes to the treatment of such patients.

Beyond rabies, the related lyssaviruses, and SARS, we now have evidence that fruit bats are the maintaining hosts for an entire spectrum of viruses that can, and in some cases do, infect humans. Among these are the related African filoviruses, Marburg and Ebola, that cause sporadic, often fatal, and highly contagious (by direct human contact) hemorrhagic disease. Then, latest but perhaps not least, there is the problem of the henipaviruses, an amalgam of Hendra and Nipah, both of which are carried by Pteropid fruit bats (literally, "flying foxes"). First detected in 1999 as a cause of fatal encephalitic (brain) disease in humans and pigs in Malaysia, Nipah virus has now caused outbreaks as far north as Bangladesh. The related Hendra virus targets horses, with the very few cases reported so far appearing in Australia. Transmission has been limited to horse handlers and veterinarians, with death resulting from febrile, flu-like, and hemorrhagic symptoms. Despite the very low incidence in humans to date, the likelihood of a fatal outcome (less than 40%) from henipavirus infections means that it is necessary to take these pathogens very seriously.

Are the henipaviruses potential pandemic pathogens?

It doesn't look like that so far and, apart from human-to-human spread, those who live in regions where bats may be carrying these viruses probably don't need to be too obsessed about the possibility that there are infected animals in the neighborhood. Though it seems that Hendra and Nipah normally infect humans after being expanded in a "multiplier" host (horses and pigs respectively), there is also evidence that people can be infected with Nipah virus in the absence of a pig intermediary. Between 2001 and 2008, some 50% of the Nipah cases in Bangladesh are thought to have resulted from human-to-human spread, though this still remained limited in extent. Transmission between people hasn't yet been seen for Hendra, but the total number of cases is miniscule. Nocturnal in their habits, flying foxes spend their day hanging upside down from the branches of trees, not uncommonly in botanical gardens. One way of isolating viruses from them is simply to spread sheets out on the ground below, then sample the droppings.

The question remains: Why are we suddenly seeing these infections? The answer is that, apart from our increasing scientific capacity for diagnosis, we don't really know. Since HIV struck, the level of infectious disease awareness and surveillance has undoubtedly improved, especially in the developing world. Global population increased fourfold from 1900 to 2000, and twofold between 1960 and 2000, with much of that growth occurring in the poorer countries of the developing world. That has led to extensive land clearance and movement into previously forested regions where bats and other wildlife live. More people means more pigs, at least in most non-Islamic countries, while increasing prosperity also leads to Western levels of meat consumption.

In wealthy nations such as Australia, where Hendra virus suddenly emerged, population increase and greater prosperity have also been accompanied by the expansion of "hobby farms," and to more relatively inexperienced people keeping "companion" horses around the periphery of the major cities. When it comes to infectious diseases and their spread, the social component may often be as important as the basic biology. A recently developed vaccine to protect horses against Hendra virus infection works well and is now available. Provided that people can be persuaded, or required, to give this vaccine to horses, there should be no further human cases.

The movie *Contagion*—which I've already mentioned as one of the more realistic and troubling fictional demonstrations of a pandemic—explores what could happen if some novel bat *henipavirus* crossed to pigs to give an infection that spreads to, and between, humans with extraordinary ease via direct contact or respiratory exposure. So far, while that scenario is certainly not impossible, it hasn't happened. Bats, pigs, and humans have lived in the same, principally tropical environments for a very long time without providing any evidence that these species cannot happily coexist. When it comes to such scenarios, it is important that quarantine authorities should be watchful, that surveillance should be adequately funded, and that we should neither overreact nor be fearful.

Is Ebola the scariest of all viruses?

It's certainly right up there. If we just think in terms of disease severity, Ebola, along with Hendra, is a terrifying pathogen. First isolated in 1976 from hemorrhagic fever cases in the Ebola

River region of the Republic of the Congo, the case fatality rate ranges from 30% to 80% (average 68%), depending on the substrain. That excludes the non-pathogenic (for humans) Ebola/ Reston variant found initially in a U.S. primate colony and isolated more recently from sick pigs in the Philippines. All natural cases of severe Ebola have occurred in Africa, or in laboratory workers who were accidentally exposed while operating under high-security conditions. Infection in the field is via contaminated body fluids and utensils rather than by aerosol. Even so, this virus is greatly feared because it can spread quickly when it first emerges, before people understand what they are dealing with.

While there were a number of fatal cases in health care workers early on, this has greatly diminished as medical professionals became increasingly aware of the disease and have had access to appropriate protective gear. The Ebola viruses also kill large apes, gorillas, and chimpanzees, and a number of experimental vaccines have been developed to protect non-human primates. Later generation variants are in an advanced stage of development and testing, but none has yet been licensed for use in people. Research scientists working with this pathogen, along with nurses and doctors in afflicted areas of Africa, are the obvious target population for a protective vaccine. Immunizing the chimps and gorillas would also be a good idea, but that isn't an easy task for these large, wild-living species. One possibility would be to use the vaccine/ bait approach that I mentioned above for rabies.

And Ebola wasn't our first experience with the filoviruses. Back in 1967, more than 30 people in Germany and Yugoslavia were infected with the closely related Marburg virus (named for the German city in which there was an outbreak), 21 of whom eventually died. Ebola and Marburg are thought to have diverged from a common ancestor several thousand years back, and both have been traced to species of fruit bats. The Marburg pathogen traveled to Europe in African green monkeys imported for the manufacture of poliomyelitis vaccine.

Though highly infectious, the fact that these two viruses are not readily transmitted via the respiratory route and that they cause such severe, hideous, hemorrhagic disease is the probable reason for the lack of wider spread within human populations. As a consequence, while any Marburg/Ebola outbreak is monitored very closely, the likelihood that either could trigger a pandemic is low, especially as the protocols for containment and the safe nursing of such cases are now well established.

What exactly is a hemorrhagic disease?

Simply put, they are diseases that cause massive, abnormal bleeding into body tissues. Some are serious and others less so. If you're traveling in a tropical location and you develop extreme malaise, a high temperature, and evidence of bleeding, it may be remotely possible that you have contracted something like Ebola hemorrhagic fever. If that's the case, you will need to be hospitalized immediately and given the best possible professional care. Pediatricians would immediately consider meningococcemia (caused by *Neisseria meningitidis*) if confronted with such symptoms in a young child. This can be treated with antibiotics, and there are vaccines available.

Especially in the absence of fever, shedding blood via a single body orifice doesn't necessarily mean that you have been infected with some horrible pathogen. If you are living in Europe or the United States and start to bleed, the likely diagnosis depends on where the blood is and on the general clinical picture. Fecal blood contamination is indicative of gastrointestinal tract problems, perhaps colon cancer. Blood in the urine could be due to kidney stones or cancer, and there are many other, less distressing causes. Bleeding gums reflect the need for a visit to the dentist. Nosebleeds afflict some more than others, and commonly result from the dehydration and dryness associated with a long flight.

Similarly, if you cough up blood, it doesn't mean that you're infected with a hemorrhagic fever virus. You've probably seen a classic movie scene where the pale eighteenth- or nineteenth-century hero or heroine coughs delicately into a linen handkerchief, then hastens to hide the telltale bright red stain from his or her lover or fond relative. As we discussed in the previous chapter, the disease is TB, and tissue damage caused by the bacteria and the host response to the infection has led to bleeding into the tissue or airways (known as localized hemorrhage) to give the blood-contaminated mucus that is coughed into the handkerchief. With TB, coughing blood can become a more frequent occurrence as the disease progresses, and it was indeed a frightening symptom in the pre-antibiotic era. Now, of course, TB can generally be treated if caught reasonably early, though we do worry about the MDR variants, as mentioned earlier.

Anyone who coughs significant amounts of fresh blood should see a doctor immediately. The best-case scenario would be some treatable bacterial infection, even if (as with TB) we may have to take antibiotics for months or more. Particularly for heavy smokers, a more frightening possibility is lung cancer. Much more immediately dangerous than either of those, however, is the possibility that coughing blood is just one symptom of an acutely febrile (high fever) hemorrhagic virus disease. In that case, the patient would be so ill that there would be much more than blood in a handkerchief to worry about.

With the true hemorrhagic fevers, a virus that is lytic for blood capillary endothelium will cause rapid vascular breakdown. The severity can range from "petechiation," small, generally purplish hemorrhages that we may first see in the skin and the mucus membranes of the eye and mouth, to the overt bleeding into tissues and from body orifices that we describe as a "hemorrhagic diathesis." Further to any direct virus-induced damage, the severity of the underlying pathology may also be compounded by the effects of various immune response cytokines and chemokines secreted during the early phase of the disease. Part of a cascade that initially functions to limit the dissemination and growth of an invading pathogen, these innate response mediators can also be associated with edema—accumulation of fluid and resultant tissue swelling—hemorrhage, and septic shock, which is again a consequence of massive vascular leakage and bleeding.

From the clinical aspect, hemorrhagic diseases are the most visually terrifying of all pathogens, which makes them ideal candidates for horror movies like *Outbreak*, *Contagion* and the 2002 British film *Twenty-Eight Days*, which postulates a pathogen that has the capacity to provoke the violent aggression and biting associated with rabies plus the hemorrhagic symptoms characteristic of the filoviruses like Ebola. Even in the absence of any fictional biting scenario, the combination of fever, petechiae (purple spots on the skin caused by broken capillaries), and severe debility provides an immediate warning to health professionals that they should take the most stringent precautions to avoid being splashed with infected blood or mucus. Even so, no highly contagious hemorrhagic fever virus has yet caused a pandemic. But there are plenty of possible contenders and, of course, we don't know what else might be out there in some wildlife reservoir. The known threats are very closely watched by the responsible organizations, like the European ECDC, the U.S. CDC, and the WHO.

Are filoviruses the main cause of hemorrhagic fevers?

No, quite the contrary, though they may be the most visually and clinically terrifying. There are lots of different types of viruses and bacteria that can cause hemorrhagic disease. When it comes to pandemic threats, however, most of these are not strong candidates, as they do not transmit readily from person to person. For instance, Weil's disease, caused by the water-borne spirochete *Leptospira icterohemorrhagiae* that grows in rat kidney tubules, is endemic worldwide and is readily cured by antibiotics. You could catch that if you fall into a freshwater canal in, say, the "low countries" of Europe. Other *Leptospira* species that can infect humans are primarily diseases of cattle, dogs, and forest-dwelling species in tropical environments. All are easily treated with drugs like streptomycin.

Then there are the hantaviruses that cause hemorrhagic fever with renal syndrome (HFRS). There is a whole range of these HFRS pathogens that first came to Western medical attention in the 1950s, during the Korean War. Living and fighting in the rural landscape, troops were exposed to an unknown enemy, the striped field mouse (*Apodemus agrarius*) that carries Korean hemorrhagic fever (KHF) virus. The usual route of exposure is by breathing dust particles that are contaminated with dried rodent urine or fecal material. Unattractive as it may seem, we breathe in stuff like that all the time. If, in fact, these viruses were carried by the common house mouse (*Mus musculus*) or by the ubiquitous urban brown rat (*Rattus norvegicus*), such infections would be much more commonplace. In any large city or old house, we often live much closer to those species than we might like to think.

Though the disease is not primarily hemorrhagic, the pulmonary syndrome (also called Navajo flu) that was first detected in the Four Corners (Colorado, New Mexico, Arizona, Utah) region of the United States is caused by another hantavirus, Sin Nombre (meaning "nameless" in Spanish). An outbreak in 2012 at Yosemite National Park led to 10 confirmed cases (with 2 deaths). The CDC issued warnings to some 10,000 summer visitors, with those who stayed in tented cabins being at greatest risk. Maintained in nature by the deer mouse (*Peromysces maniculatus*), this infection is distributed across much of North America. Human cases are fortunately rare, but more than 50% of those with clinical symptoms succumb. Deer mice are also known to be infected with a number of related viruses that do not transmit to humans.

And, while we're discussing pathogens carried by rodents, laboratory workers are occasionally infected with the arenavirus murine lymphocytic choriomeningitis virus (LCMV), which causes persistent infections in mice and hamsters. Some years back, a U.S. outbreak of severe headaches, fever, and myalgia (muscle pain) in the broader population was traced to LCMV contracted from pet hamsters that all came from one distributor. The far more severe Lassa fever arenavirus is yet another cause of acute hemorrhagic fever and is maintained in nature by the multimammate mouse (*Mastomys natalensis*) found across much of Sub-Saharan Africa. Classified (like LCMV) as an arenavirus, Lassa is distantly related to a whole spectrum of South American hemorrhagic fever viruses (Junin, Machupo, Venezuelan HFV, Bolivian HFV, Tacaribe, and so forth). All are carried by rodent species (*Calomys callosus*, for example) and, under hospital conditions where there is close contact between nurses and patients, there can be some localized person-to-person spread. In the past, it was also necessary to reinforce the message that hypodermic needles should not be used on more than one patient, but that's hardly likely to occur now when disposables are widely available and everyone is so conscious of the need to avoid the blood transmission of HIV and hepatitis C virus.

Apart from the fevers spread by exposure to pathogens excreted into the environment by other species, the Rift Valley Fever virus (*Bunyavirus*), named for the Ugandan town Bunyamwera, is a mosquito-borne infection of African cattle that causes occasional hemorrhagic disease in people. Between March and July 2009, another insect-borne *bunyavirus* emerged in China as a cause of severe febrile disease with associated thrombocytopenia. Penia is Latin for "lack of," and the thrombocytes, or platelets, are needed for normal blood clotting. Platelet deficiency is a cause of hemorrhage, and this new bunyavirus has been associated with a 30% mortality rate in clinical cases from several rural provinces of central China.

Of course, insect-borne viruses are limited by the distribution of the carrier mosquito. Geographic barriers, like oceans, can also limit the spread of such diseases, and those in cooler climates may be readily protected. We will continue that discussion in the next chapter.

The bottom line is that we simply have to live with bats, field mice, and any number of creatures. When we go out into the fields and forests, we share their world. Bats are of enormous environmental importance. They pollinate plants, move seeds and nutrients around, and keep insect numbers down. When it comes to field mice, there's no acceptable way of limiting their numbers and, in any case, who would want to wipe out any native animal? Avoiding infection with any diseases that such species carry is simply a matter of being aware and, when necessary, modifying our own behavior. And there's always the possibility of developing a vaccine for something that becomes a serious problem for us.

6

VIRUS VECTORS

What is a vector?

In the context of virus and other infections, a vector is an insect carrier of disease. What we're talking about here are living needles in the grass, like ticks, and flying needles, like mosquitoes. One of the major U.S. tire companies markets a product called "Vector," which is rather ironic because discarded tires holding pools of rainwater are favored sites for breeding mosquito larvae. Following heavy rainfalls in 2008, people living in the wetter regions of Paraguay, Brazil, and Argentina suffered severe dengue and yellow fever outbreaks. We've seen a similar situation recently in Australia with (after more than a decade of drought) flooding due to excess "La Niña" rainfall being followed by an increased incidence of the debilitating skin and joint disease caused by the mosquito-born Ross River (RRV) and Barmah Forest viruses. Horses have also been dying from encephalitis caused by Kunjin virus, which is closely related to the West Nile virus (WNV) that again came to prominence in the summer of 2012.

Although the summer was very hot and dry, there were still a large number of WNV cases. This is an intriguing example of how a "perfect storm" of weather-related events can lead to disease outbreaks. At least in some areas of the United States, the relatively mild 2011–2012 winter is thought to have favored the survival of the principal WNV vector, the mosquito *Culex pipiens*. Then, early rains set up pools of groundwater, which were not regularly flushed by further falls during the prolonged dry period. Drought also limits the availability of sites where WNV-infected birds, particularly American Robins (*Turdus migratorius*), can water, while at the same time bringing birds into contact with mosquitos. This led to a sudden upturn of cases across the country.

There is as yet no human vaccine, though several candidates are in advanced development. The best available solution—apart from using repellants or staying in screened spaces—was to use environmental spraying as a means of mosquito control. As of December 2012, the CDC recorded a total of 5,387 reported U.S. clinical cases for the calendar year, with 2,653 that showed neurological symptoms and 243 deaths. At least half the known cases were in Texas. Also, this virus causes human viremia, and WNV was detected in some 597 blood donors, who presumably felt fine when they presented themselves, though 16% went on to develop clinical signs. The contaminated blood was, of course, discarded and not used, an improvement over the situation in 2002, when 23 WNV cases were linked back to blood transfusion.

What is WNV, and has it been around for very long?

You probably won't have any childhood memories of WNV if you were born before 1999, when this disease was first diagnosed in New York City. That initial U.S. outbreak was first picked up by the sudden, increased incidence of human neurological disease and by the fact that, right at the same time, crows were falling from the sky and exotic birds, such as flamingoes, were dying in New York's Bronx Zoo. Over the next 5 years, traveling in a mosquito/bird (especially robins, finches, crows, and magpies) transmission cycle, the disease spread across the U.S. continent to California, up into Canada and down through

Mexico to South America. Until 2011, the CDC recorded about 30,000 human cases, with a 4% incidence of mortality in those who showed any obvious clinical symptoms.

Indeed, the incidence of neurological disease, or WNV-induced meningoencephalitis—the potentially lethal infection of the brain and its surrounding membranes—is generally low. Most who are bitten by an infected mosquito—including 84% of the viremic blood donors mentioned above—suffer only a subclinical or mild, flu-like illness. That could be how the WNV came to the United States in 1999, though it is also possible that it was introduced in an infected mosquito holed up somewhere on a commercial flight that originated in Israel or the southern regions of Russia, where the disease was then active. Apart from an infected, asymptomatic, human traveler, a further possibility is that it was introduced in the blood of an imported, or free-flying, bird, though the latter does not fit the profile for any known avian migratory pathway.

People aren't important for the survival of WNV in nature. We are what epidemiologists call "incidental" hosts, and the same is probably true for horses, which can also die from WNV infection. There is a vaccine for horses, reflecting that the less stringent requirement for safety testing makes it much easier, and infinitely cheaper, to develop products that are intended solely for veterinary use. The greatest losers as a consequence of the WNV incursion have been birds. When the virus first reached California, there was a massive die-off in the iconic yellow tailed magpie population, which had been chosen by the local Audubon Society members as the state bird for that year.

WNV infects birds, horses, and humans—does it also multiply in mosquitoes?

Yes, WNV is what's called an arbovirus, or arthropod-borne virus, which means that, while such pathogens multiply in the tissues of various warm-blooded vertebrates like us, they also replicate in the salivary glands of mosquitoes, with huge numbers of virions accumulating in the insects' extracellular spaces. Other arboviruses have a somewhat similar life cycle in ticks, which—unlike mosquitoes, where only the females transmit the infection—do not discriminate on the basis of sex. And, while the adaptive immune systems of the higher vertebrates—the birds and mammals—generally eliminate the virus within 6 to 10 days, the only thing likely to terminate such infections in a tick or mosquito is the death of the arthropod host.

Tick-borne viruses are the cause of louping ill, a fatal encephalitis of sheep and grouse in the United Kingdom, and the closely related human diseases Russian spring/summer encephalitis and Central European encephalitis. After a long, hard winter, a picnic on the grass is a true delight, but ticks may be lurking and a personal catastrophe can follow. The tick-borne Kyasanur Forest disease is known to infect some 100–500 people annually in India, causing a hemorrhagic disease with a morbidity—or illness rate—of about 2–4%. A very minor problem in North America, Powassan virus has been responsible for some 20 known clinical cases. Clearly, however, the tick-borne viruses are even less likely to be pandemic candidates than those carried by mosquitoes. When it comes to any intercontinental transfer, the likelihood that some global traveler with a subclinical infection might encounter an appropriate blood-sucking tick would have to be very low!

All the above viruses, whether spread via tick or mosquito vectors, are further classified as flaviviruses, a large group containing many "orphans" that are not known to cause any human or veterinary disease. Among the pathogens, Australians will be familiar with Murray Valley encephalitis virus and Kunjin virus, both of which are closely related to WNV. And those living in the Asia/Pacific region should have been vaccinated against the worst of these neuropathology-causing arboviruses, Japanese B encephalitis virus (JEV), which is largely maintained in a mosquito/pig life cycle.

Of great concern are the four serotypes of dengue virus that replicate only in humans and insects and cause "break-bone" fever in Africa, the Western Pacific and Southeast Asia regions, the Caribbean, and the Southern United States. No bones are actually broken; it just feels that way. The symptoms include fever, muscle and joint pain, and a measles-like rash. A further manifestation is the much less common dengue hemorrhagic fever (DHF), which is generally a problem in children who have recovered from one strain of dengue virus and are then infected with a second variant in the following year. For reasons that are still incompletely understood, this can lead to low platelet counts, blood and serum leakage, and the development of what is called dengue shock syndrome. While many children died early on, clinical outcomes have improved dramatically with the skilled application of supportive—basically fluid reconstitution—therapy, and most now survive. Cases of DHF were also seen in young Americans who spent significant time serving with the military, or President John F. Kennedy's Peace Corps, in endemic regions. There are currently no effective vaccines to protect against any of the dengue serotypes, though such products have been under development for decades.

And we've barely mentioned the "big daddy" of the flaviviruses, the prototype yellow fever virus (YFV). *Flavi* is Latin for "yellow," reflecting that, apart from fever and general malaise, the primary symptom is jaundice. Though there's been a good vaccine for more than half a century, this disease is still a problem in parts of Africa and South America. The existence of a "maintaining" sylvatic cycle in wildlife, poverty, and the lack of a proper medical infrastructure means that there are still about 30,000–40,000 deaths and 200,000 cases per year, mostly in West Africa.

What exactly is yellow fever virus?

Basically, YFV enters via the skin, travels around the body in the blood, and destroys the liver. Starting with high fever and flu-like symptoms, there is a rapid progression to bleeding and pronounced jaundice of the skin and mucus membranes. This is due to the presence of blood-borne bilirubin, a molecule that is produced when "effete"—meaning past their use-by date and no longer effective—red blood cells (RBCs.) are eliminated. Following the destruction of "old" red cells, a physiological process that goes on all the time, the iron-containing heme complex (the RBC oxygen carrier) gives rise to bilirubin, which is normally conjugated with glucuronic acid in the liver, then oxidized and eliminated in the bile as stercobilin and urobilin. The minor bile ducts drain to the gallbladder, located behind the liver. Stercobilin is responsible for the characteristic brown pigment of feces, while some urobilin is resorbed into the blood and excreted in the urine, giving the familiar straw to yellow color. Jaundice (yellowing) means that there is an excess of these breakdown products in the blood. Possible causes include virus- or toxin-induced damage to the liver cells; the excessive breakdown of red blood cells (malaria, rhesus disease in the newborn); or blockage of the common bile duct that carries the bilirubin breakdown products from the gallbladder to the intestine.

Yellow fever, also called "yellow jack," devastated tropical military and colonial expeditions over the centuries, from Alexander the Great through the Napoleonic wars, and aborted the initial 1880s effort by Ferdinand de Lesseps to cut a canal through the Isthmus of Panama. Then, in 1904, the Americans took over the canal-building enterprise. Their ultimate success reflects the fact that they controlled yellow fever. U.S. Army medical officer Walter Reed confirmed the idea (advanced by Cuban physician and scientist Carlos Finlay) that YFV is spread by the *Aedes egypti* mosquito (see Figure 6.1). Reed and William Gorgas introduced a strict regime of mosquito control by eliminating sources of standing water where the mosquito "wrigglers" breed, or by covering such water with a film of kerosene. At the same time, these measures reduced the damage done by another mosquito-borne infection, the protozoan malaria parasite.

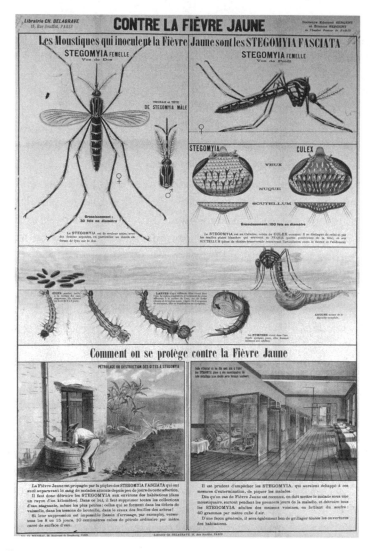

Figure 6.1. You don't need to read French to see that this yellow fever poster advocates sleeping under bed nets and pouring kerosene on the top of open water barrels to stop the mosquito wrigglers (larvae) from breathing. Believed to be from 1907, donated to the National Library of Medicine by Drs. Edmond and Étienne Sergent of the Institut Pasteur, Paris.

From the Historical Images Archive of the National Library of Medicine.

Prior to 1882, YFV caused outbreaks in New York and Boston, and the disease remained active for much longer in the American South. By the end of the 1878 epidemic year, more than 5,000 had died in Memphis and 4,600 in New Orleans, with the lower Mississippi River valley recording at least 20,000 deaths. Even now, Southern cities maintain very effective mosquito control—environmental spraying—programs through the hotter months. Perhaps the fact that there had been less of a historical problem with insect-borne pathogens in Texas explains why many municipalities came rather late to this mechanism for limiting the 2012 WNV outbreak.

We do have a yellow fever vaccine, though: the very effective 17D yellow fever vaccine, developed in New York City during the 1930s at the old Rockefeller Institute—now Rockefeller University—by South African–born scientist Max Theiler. This earned him the 1951 Nobel Prize for Physiology or Medicine, the only one to date given directly for the development of a vaccine, though John Enders, Tom Weller, and Fred Robbins (1954), Baruch Blumberg (1976), and Harald zur Hausen (2008) were honored for basic science discoveries and developments that led ultimately to vaccines against poliomyelitis, hepatitis B, and human papilloma virus, respectively.

What do we know about the global movements of arboviruses?

It's a long story and we don't know all the details. The U.S. WNV story has shown us quite recently that such viruses do indeed jump ocean barriers. As summarized by the WHO, only nine countries had experienced severe dengue epidemics before 1970, but the disease is now endemic in more than 100 nations in Africa, the Americas, the Eastern Mediterranean, Southeast Asia, and the Western Pacific. To me, that sounds like "vector" jet planes moving infected people. Long before mass air travel, YFV clearly had been established in both Africa and the Americas. This disease is not in Southeast Asia, for example, and YFV likely reached the Americas in sixteenth-century slave ships. Also, the north/south distribution of any arbovirus will obviously depend on the geographic range of the particular mosquito strain.

Dramatic illustrations of recent spread come from the alphaviruses, a different class of mosquito-borne arboviruses. Americans may be familiar with the Eastern and Western equine encephalitis viruses, though these are not the cause of much current concern. What is being watched more closely is the subgroup of alphaviruses that cause the syndrome described as epidemic polyarthritis with rash. These include RRV in Australia and, more dramatically, Chikungunya virus out of Africa, which is on the move.

Known clinically since the eighteenth century and first isolated in Tanzania in 1953, Chikungunya means "that which bends up" in the Makonda language, giving some idea of the associated human suffering. Maintained in people and other primates, this virus, which is now prevalent in Thailand, Indonesia, Malaysia, and Irian Jaya (West Papua), also caused some 200+ generally mild cases in northern Italy in 2007. A great deal of current effort is focused on making a good human vaccine. Though limited in northern range by the distribution of the two principal mosquito vectors, *Aedes aegyptii* and *Aedes albopictus*, the extent of Chikungunya spread certainly fulfills the WHO influenza pandemic alert criteria discussed in Chapter 2.

Do mosquitoes and ticks really carry needles?

Kind of: in fact, the mouthparts of both are made of multiple bits, including the mandibles and maxillae. That describes our jawbones, of course, though the boneless arthropods use the tough chitin that forms their exoskeleton to make such strong structures. In mosquitoes, the paired mandibles and maxillae form the needle-like stylets that breach the tough skin barrier and, with the aid of tissue-dissolving enzymes and anticoagulant proteins present in the virus-laden saliva, allow them to feed on our blood while holding the insect in place. The tick does much the same thing, with multiple, harpoon-like barbs on an inserted structure called the hypostoma, aided by a secreted, cement-like substance that forms a tight attachment.

That's why, when removing a tick, it's best to use tweezers or some similar tool to gently pry away the mouthparts. Then keep the tick in a plastic bag in the refrigerator so, if you do develop a fever, it can be ground up in a homogenizer (by a lab technician, not in your kitchen) and tested for a possible pathogen. In the United States particularly, what you will watch closely for over the next month or more is the spreading rash caused by the spirochete *Borrrelia burgdorfei*, the cause of Lyme disease. This infection has been reported from every continent except Antarctica, though there is no hard evidence that it is in Australia. People can also develop hemolytic anemia due to infection with tick-borne *Babesia* (protozoa) species, especially if they have had their spleen removed. And ticks also carry bacteria like *Anaplasma* and *Ehrlichia* that cause human fevers and malaise. All these diseases can be treated with antibiotics.

What are the pandemic risks when it comes to these vectored viruses?

While there is no obvious way that an insect-borne virus could, like the influenza A viruses, cause a rapidly spreading, global pandemic, the dengue experience over the past 40 years tells us that they do get around. Clearly, the distribution of such pathogens will always be restricted by the geographic range of both their maintaining hosts—humans for dengue, birds for WNV—and their arthropod vectors. Even so, those living in more temperate latitudes should not be too complacent. Both YFV and malaria struck as far north as the St. Lawrence River in the eighteenth and nineteenth centuries, and 2012 saw cases of WNV encephalitis in Maine, Minnesota, Quebec, and Ontario.

The quarantine authorities would no doubt detect any ticks carried by imported livestock, racehorses, and the like, though it's always possible that an infected tick could cross the oceans attached to some smuggled bird or small mammal. Even so, the likelihood that a viremic vertebrate might provide a blood meal for an appropriate vector tick in a new landscape would seem very remote. Of course, that's much less improbable for any mosquito-borne pathogen, as illustrated by the WNV invasion of the United States. Over the course of 5 years, the CDC documented the spread of WNV across the country in a bird-mosquito life cycle, and much the same thing (though we don't know the maintaining host) has happened with RRV in Australia. Both infections are now permanently endemic across these two large continental landmasses.

Like our early ancestors, Chikungunyah virus has moved into southern Europe and around the Indian Ocean rim to Southeast Asia. It hasn't yet reached Australia, though RRV and the closely related Barmah Forest virus cause very similar symptoms. The appropriate mosquito vectors for Chikungunya and for Japanese encephalitis virus (JEV) are in Australia, and we have seen the occasional JEV case in the hot, tropical north. A great fear with these mosquito-borne viruses is that anthropogenic global warming will lead to their migration away from the equator and to higher altitudes. We're already seeing that with malaria.

As illustrated by the 2012 WNV experience, the damage done by all mosquito-borne viruses can be limited by environmental spraying, but, as this is an add-on for stretched municipal and state budgets where the likelihood of such infections is generally low, there will be no contingency funds set aside. Also, since the inexpensive DDT was outlawed for environmental use because of the damage it does to the shells of bird's eggs, the cost of spraying in poorer countries can be prohibitive. That's part of the reason that some 500,000 children still die each year from malaria. Spraying with DDT inside houses, together with the use of DDT-impregnated bed nets, however, has proven to be both effective and environmentally safe. And for the arboviruses (though not malaria), making appropriate human vaccines, if the economic and medical justifications were deemed sufficient, should be a relatively straightforward task. We already have licensed human products for flaviviruses like YFV and JEV, and veterinary vaccines are given to protect valuable horses from WNV and the Eastern and Western equine encephalitis alphaviruses.

7

SINGLE-HOST HUMAN PATHOGENS

Is an infection that is already widespread in humans likely to cause a pandemic?

As discussed previously, that really gets down to a matter of terminology. The influenza A viruses that emerge as a consequence of genetic reassortment, perhaps between viruses circulating in us and in birds, are referred to as pandemic strains. On the other hand, a new escape variant that causes a global "seasonal" epidemic as a consequence of mutation within a currently circulating influenza A virus is not accorded that status. The distinction is legitimate in the public health sense, as a novel pandemic virus is likely to be both more unique and less predictable. Even so, while those who work with variant noroviruses are in much the same situation that we confront with seasonal influenza, they speak of novel pandemic strains.

What are noroviruses?

You might be more familiar with the term if your cruising holiday had been ruined because everyone came down with vomiting and diarrhea. A ship, even if large and well stabilized, is the last place anyone wants to be in such circumstances.

But the reason we don't normally think of noroviruses as pandemic viruses is that, though the disease they cause may be transiently discomforting, it is rarely fatal. The norovirus dynamic can also operate in hospitals, or in any other situation where large numbers of people are essentially confined.

The term *norovirus* comes from the prototype "Norwalk agent"—called for the town in Ohio where the first recognized outbreak occurred. The noroviruses are now known to cause more than 70% of gastroenteritis (stomach flu) outbreaks in the United States and there are some 40 different types, with the GII4 strains showing the most troubling rate of mutations. Those working with the noroviruses consider that five global GII4 pandemics occurred over the past 15 years, all of them resulting in substantial absenteeism and consequential economic loss. They certainly qualify as pandemic or "seasonal epidemic" pathogens by the WHO influenza criteria for spread but, again, they don't fulfill the public idea of "very bad infection."

Of course, the fact that we are marginally aware of the noroviruses would change rapidly if they mutated to greater virulence—which could happen. The noroviruses belong to the calicivirus family and, as discussed later in this book, a lethal hemorrhagic disease caused by a virulent rabbit calicivirus was spread deliberately as a pest control strategy in Australia. Fortunately, the caliciviruses do tend to be very species-specific, and the rabbit calicivirus was first tested extensively to ensure that it would not infect indigenous wildlife. Even so, these viruses are incredibly infectious, and the development of antiviral therapeutics that target key elements in the GII4-strain replication pathways would seem urgent. There should be a ready market for such drugs now, at least in the tourism industry.

Are the noroviruses our only concern when it comes to the virus diarrheas?

No, especially when it comes to young children. Various strains of rotavirus are endemic globally and are the most common cause of GI tract infections and severe diarrhea for babies. The big danger here is dehydration, with as many as 450,000 infants still dying annually from rotavirus infections in the developing countries. Nonetheless, the mortality rate has been greatly reduced by the introduction of simple, cheap procedures for oral rehydration. And after a rocky start—due to an elevated incidence of bowel intussusception associated with an early product—the WHO now regards the currently available, live-attenuated (like oral polio) rotavirus vaccines as safe and recommends that they be included in routine immunization schedules for all young children.

What is intussusception?

That happens when one length of bowel "telescopes" back into another to cause a blockage of the GI tract. The condition is not uncommon in very young children, but the original rotavirus vaccine did seem to be associated with an increased incidence of the problem.

Are there other ways of protecting against these viruses?

Just common sense: the best protection against any GI tract infection is to practice rigorous hand hygiene. Another good habit is to minimize the extent of hand-to-face, hand-to-nose, and hand-to-eye contact. Alcohol wipes and detergent may not be very effective with the noroviruses, whose outer coat lacks the lipids that are damaged by such chemicals. The prominent, wall-mounted *Purell* hand sanitizers work better and are increasingly a feature of at-risk institutions everywhere.

In the event of becoming infected, the most important thing to do (apart from seeing a doctor) is to avoid dehydration by maintaining a high fluid intake. In short, drink as much water as you can hold and, if available, add "physiological" salts (see last chapter) to keep your blood in balance. That is particularly important for the very young and the elderly. A simple test for dehydration is to pinch a fold of skin on the back of the fore-arm—to see whether the skin "springs back" or creates a "little tent," an indication of severe dehydration. Do the "pinch test" and measure your normal "baseline" while feeling well, perhaps when waiting to board a flight to some exotic destination. And avoid the very dehydrating consequences of excess alcohol consumption at high altitudes. Even with precautions, if you're traveling in the developing world, all bets are off if you suddenly suffer severe GI tract symptoms, diarrhea, fever, and headache, perhaps with associated rose-colored skin spots. The cause could be cholera or typhoid and you will need immediate antibiotic treatment.

Apart from the hemorrhagic viruses, are cholera and typhoid the main causes of skin spots?

No, especially when we're talking about kids. Though endemic rather than potential pandemic problems, there are many fever-associated childhood rashes, or exanthemas. Bacterial infections, like scarlet fever (*Streptococcus*) and staphylococcal scalded skin syndrome are readily treated with antibiotics. The "R" component of the MMR vaccine protects against rubella (German measles). We also have a vaccine for chicken pox (varicella, Herpes zoster), which is, again, disseminated around the body (including to the skin) in the lymph and blood after first entering via the oropharynx. This virus "hides out" in the dorsal root ganglia (cumulated nerve bodies) of the spinal cord where, as immune control fails with age, it can emerge again, or reactivate, to cause a painful condition, shingles, in the elderly. Then there are no vaccines for the generally mild early childhood conditions, erythema infectiousum (parvovirus B19) and roseola infantum (human herpesvirus 6 and 7). Parvovirus B19 causes a "slapped cheeks" appearance in little kids, but it can be a major problem for the developing fetus if it crosses the placenta in an infected mother.

Is measles something that we should still be worried about?

Like polio, measles is one virus that we should be able to eradicate, as it is genetically stable and persists only in humans. One problem is that it spreads very readily. Another is that significant numbers of parents in the developed world are denying their offspring access to the vaccines that protect against the common infectious diseases of childhood. As a consequence, we see occasional school outbreaks where, for instance, an unvaccinated teenager vacationing with his parents in a developing country contracts the disease and brings it back home. Then, there are also instances where an infected European child has reintroduced this disease to a third world country that had gained the upper hand as a result of a major measles eradication campaign.

Measles is both extremely infectious and a bad pathogen. It can be lethal, particularly in the undernourished and the immunocompromised, including those who are undergoing cancer chemotherapy or have untreated HIV/AIDS. As with polio, the measles virus enters via the nose or mouth to grow initially in the mucosal epithelium of the upper respiratory tract and oropharynx (back of the throat). The attenuated vaccine virus stops right there and does not spread further, but fully virulent measles virus goes on to cause viremia. The characteristic Koplik spots are seen only after the virus has disseminated to the skin via the blood. This acute phase is normally terminated within a week or two by the virus-specific immune response and, once the virus is eliminated, recovery soon follows. But that isn't the totality of the measles story.

The danger is that the viremic phase can lead to this pathogen invading sites like the middle ear, the lung, the kidney, and the brain. About 1:1,000 of those infected develop encephalitis, which can be fatal. And there are long-term sequelae. At least some cases of the debilitating, chronic lung condition bronchiectasis are thought to result from damage associated with measles and/or whooping cough in childhood. Another potential danger is the terrible, though fortunately rare, neurological condition subacute sclerosing panencephalitis (SSPE). In these cases, the measles virus "hides out" in the brain as a defective form that can reemerge and cause damage years later. Characteristically, a happy and active teenager suddenly goes into a coma and dies. Infectious disease professionals were universally delighted as the emerging epidemiological evidence indicated that the measles vaccine had consigned SSPE to the history of medicine; but if parents won't vaccinate their children, this may not be the case.

Are there any other kinds of GI tract infections?

Indeed; so many that we can't cover the entire list. There is a whole spectrum of enteroviruses and adenoviruses, for example, that are known to cause GI, respiratory, renal, and even some brain infections. But there is a further, major human pathogen that enters via the GI tract and causes severe disease: hepatitis A. Hepatitis A virus is both spread under conditions of poor hygiene and is one of the infections that we contract from eating uncooked oysters harvested in an estuary where raw human sewage is being discharged. Filter feeders that process large amounts of seawater over their gills, oysters simply concentrate hepatitis A virus from the environment.

Is there a good hepatitis vaccine?

Yes and no: we do have effective commercial vaccines that protect against hepatitis (Hep) A, B, D and (very likely) E, though HepC continues to defeat us in this regard. These different hepatitis viruses are only related by the fact that each causes liver pathology of varying duration and severity. The HepA–E letters are just another classification system that broadly reflects when these viruses were first identified.

Though widely distributed through, particularly, the poorer countries, HepA generally causes a self-limiting disease that rarely goes on to cause chronic problems. The HepB vaccines protect against both B and D, and there are major efforts to immunize all children in those areas of the developing world where both HepA and HepB are prevalent. And it's a wise precaution for more adventurous travelers to be immunized against HepB, especially those who might be open to random sexual encounters. Because HepA is so infectious and readily contracted via the alimentary route, the HepA vaccine is mandatory for all tourists visiting exotic locations, no matter how impeccable they may be when it comes to personal hygiene. Can you ever be quite sure how, and by whom, your food has been handled? Contracting HepA can really spoil your vacation, though you will likely recover before too long.

Like HepA, HepE causes a self-limiting disease—meaning that it's effectively controlled by the adaptive immune response. Perhaps heralding future trends, a HepE vaccine produced and approved for human use in China is now at the point of being marketed. Because this disease mainly afflicts the poor—70,000 die annually—there was no commercial incentive for Western companies to make such a product. Unlike the other hepatitis viruses we're discussing here, HepE is carried by pigs and is not maintained primarily in humans. Transmitted like HepA via oral/fecal contamination, HepE infection is debilitating in the short term, and mortality rates can be as high as 1–2%, with that increasing to more than 5% in the elderly. Women of reproductive age are primary targets for vaccination, as this virus can cause abortion and fetal (and occasional maternal) death when contracted in the second or third trimester.

But there's no immediate prospect of a vaccine against HepC. Like yellow fever, HepC virus is a flavivirus, though the needle that transmits this infection is not mounted on a mosquito but on a hypodermic syringe wielded by human hands. What further separates HepC from all the genetically stable, arthropod-borne flaviviruses is that, as is the case for HIV, it persists within infected people via a mechanism that involves the constant selection of immune escape variants.

This difference between the infinitely variable HepC and the more conserved insect-borne flaviviruses likely reflects that, while both need to be at high concentrations in the blood, the transfer of HepC infection via a contaminated syringe needle is an essentially passive process. On the other hand, the very demanding life cycle that enables a naturally transmitted pathogen to replicate in both vertebrate (bird, pig, human) and arthropod (mosquito or tick) tissues may allow little possibility for change.

Are HepB and HepC the most dangerous of the hepatitis viruses?

They are, and there's a sad story about HepB that, nonetheless, provides a further example of how modern science protects us. Back in the dark days of 1942, the U.S. Army inadvertently injected thousands of troops with a batch of yellow fever vaccine that contained human serum contaminated with the as yet undiscovered HepB virus. The net result was acute illness, followed by long-term health consequences for many veterans.

By the 1970s, we had tests to screen for the presence of blood-borne HepB, but physicians were still seeing a high incidence of liver disease (called at that time "hepatitis non-A, non-B") associated with transfusion and the administration of blood products like clotting factors (for hemophiliacs). By the time HepC was identified in the 1980s, some 300,000 Americans had contracted the virus as a consequence of receiving contaminated blood. Since then, transmission has continued in the United States via the sharing of infected needles in the drug-injecting population. The same is true for HepB, though HepB also spreads as a consequence of both heterosexual and MSM (men who have sex with men) activity. That can occur with HepC, though it is much less common.

In the absence of a vaccine, there are currently about 18,000 new HepC infections each year in the United States. Somewhere between 2.7 and 3.9 million people are chronic carriers, and about 12,000 die annually from liver failure. At least

180 million people are infected worldwide, with the numbers in Egypt being particularly high because of the reuse of needles in an early vaccination campaign. The incidence of persistent infection, and thus chronic hepatitis, runs in the 25–35% range for those who contract the disease.

Over the years, some have been treated successfully with a protracted course (enduring as long as nearly a year) of pegylated type 1 interferon and the antiviral *Ribavirin*, but this is very expensive and far from universally successful. The big hope with HepC lies in newly developed drugs, two of which (both HepC virus protease inhibitors) have recently been approved by the FDA for human use. Perhaps, given that HepC is transmitted only by needle spread, it may be possible to eliminate this virus by aggressive therapy. That would be a first for humanity. The only viruses that we have eradicated so far (smallpox in humans, rinderpest in cattle) were disposed of by a combination of intelligent management and vaccination.

Why is chronic hepatitis so dangerous?

The answer is twofold: liver infections can lead to cancer and/or terminal liver failure. The problem is that the host immune response keeps trying to do its job and get rid of the persistent virus. The net consequence is the continued presence of all sorts of invading WBCs (immune T cells, macrophages, and so forth) that secrete various cytokines and chemokines and cause chronic inflammation. This combination of ongoing virus and immune cell damage leads to cirrhosis, where functional hepatic cells (hepatocytes) are replaced by connective tissue. The end result is a scarred, hardened, and progressively dysfunctional liver.

This continuing inflammatory pathology and consequent cirrhosis cause the liver cells to proliferate as the organ tries to compensate. Every cell division carries with it the possibility of mutational change and, especially under such physiologically unfavorable conditions, the transition to cancer, namely hepatocellular carcinoma (HCC). Patients often die within a year of diagnosis. The HCC problem has traditionally been most severe in countries that have a high incidence of HepB infection, and the HepB vaccine, which has been available in various formulations since the 1980s, was the first effective human anti-cancer vaccine. Now persistent HepC has also emerged as a major cancer risk factor, and it is currently the leading reason for liver transplants in the United States.

Of course, excess alcohol consumption can also lead to cirrhosis and HCC, though most cases are virus-associated. Drinking is clearly a terrible idea for anyone with chronic HepB or HepC infections, but ethanol isn't the sole cancer-inducing co-factor for HepB carriers. Continued high-risk behavior can lead to super-infection with HepD, a "subviral satellite" that can only multiply in the presence of HepB. Thought to have originated from a category of plant viruses called viroids, HepD uses some of the HBV proteins in its outer coat. Co-infection with HepD is associated with more severe hepatitis, and the enhanced development of chronic liver cirrhosis and HCC in HepB carriers.

Is it safe to have a blood transfusion?

Yes, without any doubt if you're living in a society that has a high-quality medical system. You can be sure that the blood supply has been checked for the presence of HepB, HepC, HIV, and anything else that might be present in the circulation (for example, WNV in the United States). The estimated risk of contracting HIV in the United Kingdom as a consequence of receiving contaminated blood is calculated at around one in 5 million, a level that's statistically almost nonexistent. Crossing the street is infinitely more dangerous. No medical procedure is totally without risk, but blood transfusion is among the safest. In addition, checking that blood donors are in good health minimizes the possibility that they might be incubating some other infection that causes viremia.

In the case of a surgical or trauma emergency in a region where there are serious concerns about the integrity of the blood supply, the NIH advises that blood transfusion should only be used as a last resort. Often it's possible to stabilize the patient with commercially produced plasma expanders with, for the most severe cases, rapid evacuation by air to an advanced medical center. Oil and gas workers who work in remote, difficult, and sometimes dangerous situations are generally insured to cover such emergencies. Except for the most prominent and at-risk among us, the U.S. president for example, it's not feasible to travel with our own matched, clean blood supply. A great deal of current research is directed at developing blood substitutes to improve cost, safety, and availability.

Even when there is the possibility of exposure to contaminated blood, the relative risk of infection varies greatly and is calculated at around 30% for hepatitis B, 3% for hepatitis C, and 0.3% for HIV. A highly unlikely scenario is the possibility of being splashed with blood when helping someone who has been in a fight or is bleeding profusely following a motor vehicle accident. Should that happen, it's important to wear glasses and gloves if available, wash off any blood with soap and water (or disinfectant), and then seek medical advice if the disease status of the victim is unknown. Though it was not the case in the distant past, we're all accustomed to the fact that our dentist, for example, will be wearing gloves and a protective mask.

Are any of these single-host human pathogens likely to cause pandemics?

Well, novel noroviruses do and will continue to cause regular pandemics, at least if we accept the definition as being global spread. However, so long as they are not associated with more than transient and inconvenient infections, we are not too bothered by them. Diseases like poliomyelitis and measles are extremely infectious, but there's only a general risk if we drop our vaccination coverage to the level where "herd immunity" no longer prevents virus spread. That can be in the 80–90% range, but then only those who are unvaccinated will be vulnerable. That's why it is so important to maintain a high level of vaccine protection in children.

With regard to the various hepatitis viruses, any occurrence is more likely to be at the outbreak, rather than the epidemic or pandemic level. Even so, particularly with such blood-borne and/or sexually transmitted diseases, there can be isolated "islands" or even "continents" of human population where the infection is yet to take hold. If, as occurred following the collapse of the Soviet Union, the security of the blood supply is compromised due to social disruption or the withdrawal of funding, diseases like HepC could rapidly become a problem, particularly for high-risk groups such as hemophiliacs. In short, while probably not the stuff of future pandemics, the known hepatitis viruses remain real health threats that merit continued monitoring.

8

HIV/AIDS

Is HIV still a concern?

That depends a lot on how and where we live. The current situation for HIV is a bit like that discussed above for the HepC virus in that, while HIV is active in every nation on the planet, the great majority of human beings (99.5%) remain uninfected, a figure that falls to less than 80% in some regions of Sub-Saharan Africa. The acquired immune deficiency syndrome (AIDS), the ultimate consequence of contracting HIV, is less widespread than the virus in the sense that, where anti-HIV drugs are available and affordable, most infected people are able to function and live something like a normal life span. But those with HIV are forced to gulp a lot of pills. Some are sick often, there is a greater risk of fatal cardiovascular disease, and a few develop bizarre lipodystrophies (oddly distributed accumulations of fat).

There can be absolutely no doubt that the best approach to HIV is to take every precaution against being infected in the first place. That's especially true for people living in the poorer countries where no more than 25% of those with HIV have access to drugs and, with the current financial uncertainties, there's no guarantee that the various programs that help to sustain even this level of access will continue indefinitely. Regrettably, that decline is already beginning. The resources made available by various governments (the United States is the largest supporter) and foundations to the Global Fund to Fight AIDS, Tuberculosis and Malaria have been severely impacted. There have, however, been some extraordinary individual contributions. At the January 2012 World Economic Forum in Davos, Bill Gates donated $750 million of his own money to the Global Fund to Fight AIDS, Tuberculosis and Malaria.

In fact, if Americans need a reason to feel good about themselves in these difficult times, they might think about the support given by their fellow citizens and national government to the alleviation of these terrible diseases. Initiated in 2008 during the administration led by George W. Bush, the drugs supplied via the U.S. President's Emergency Plan for AIDS Relief (PEPFAR) made a very important contribution. And U.S. taxpayers should also consider the fantastic job done for the health of all the world's citizens by federal agencies like the National Institutes of Health (NIH) and the Centers for Disease Control and Prevention (CDC). Given that these diseases are global problems, such activities also function to provide a measure of forward defense.

Can what's happening now with HIV/AIDS be described as a pandemic?

Yes, that's what most would think. Even though HIV is long established on every continent except Antarctica, it does continue to spread. For example, about 350,000–450,000 completely innocent children are thought to have contracted the infection in 2010, and the number of AIDS deaths in that year ranged from 1.6 to 1.9 million. Perhaps the best description for AIDS is as a persisting or chronic pandemic, though I'm not sure that word usage is acceptable to all epidemiologists.

Is there any improvement in the AIDS situation?

Yes, the infection rate is generally falling in the most affected developing countries. We've known about AIDS since 1981; by

1983, the virus that causes this lethal, chronic wasting disease had been discovered. During that time, more than 30 million have died, while another 34 million are currently living with HIV. An encouraging sign is that the number of new cases each year has dropped, from 3.5 million in 1996 to around 2.6 million in 2009. Part of the decrease reflects that nations like South Africa, where some senior politicians were not acknowledging HIV as the cause of AIDS early on, now accept that incontestable reality and, as a consequence, are facilitating both appropriate publicity and greater access to preventive measures and therapies. Regrettably, they had been influenced by some senior scientist "deniers," who were abetted by irresponsible journalists in what were once regarded as respectable newspapers.

From the outset of the AIDS pandemic, we learned from experience in countries like Senegal, where all the leadership groups (including the Islamic clerics) got together to promote appropriate protective measures, that it is always better to face than to deny reality. Australia, for example, had an enormously effective TV advertisement with a black-robed, skeletal "grim reaper" delivering a bowling ball to "skittle" people of all ages and descriptions. Many of those depicted were, in fact, quite safe. Even so, while more than a little over the top, this horror scenario gained the attention of everyone and augmented strong efforts within the gay community (the group in greatest danger) to get the word out on what needed to be done. That, plus national leadership from key medical professionals, a switched-on federal health minister (Neal Blewett), and "judgment free" mobile clinics ensured that the spread of the disease was greatly diminished in those who were most vulnerable. A key component was the ready availability of condoms and clean needle exchange programs in areas frequented by at-risk people.

In the United States, opposition from various conservative groups has continued to limit the application of such simple, direct approaches and the incidence of new cases (35,000–40,000 per year) remains higher than it should be. The lesson is that, when faced with a spreading infectious disease, the political and public health approach needs to be both evidence-based and pragmatic. Fortunately, the difficulty that some have in dealing with the realities of sexually transmitted diseases and the behavior of what many regard as a dysfunctional, drug-injecting underclass does not extend to respiratory infections, our main risk when it comes to pandemics. Everyone, no matter how moral or amoral, how worthy or unworthy, how rich or poor, has to breathe!

Where did this virus come from, and why didn't we see AIDS before 1981?

Sequence analysis of the AIDS virus by Beatrice Hahn and colleagues at the University of Alabama, Birmingham, and elsewhere has established very clearly that the "parent" of the predominant HIV-1 virus (group M or main) originated from a simian immunodeficiency virus (SIV) that infects chimpanzees (*Pan troglodytes troglodytes*) in Central Africa. Initially, this was thought to be a mild, inapparent infection of chimps, though it is now known that it can also be lethal for them, our closest relatives. Other, less common HIV-1 strains look to have come from lowland gorillas (*Gorilla gorilla*) while HIV-2, which has, to date, been substantially confined to Africa, is a virus of sooty mangabeys (*Cercocybus atys atys*).

How did these viruses make the transfer from chimps, gorillas, and monkeys into people? One possibility is that, with the availability of hypodermic syringes and needles, "traditional" healers injected ground-up primate tissues directly into humans. This type of practice isn't restricted to Africa, though sheep rather than monkeys are the preferred source of the animal material used in, for example, Swiss cell-therapy clinics. Apart from the fact that there is no scientific basis for such treatments, given that the prototype prion disease is sheep scrapie (as discussed later), it would be sensible to avoid them. The "mad cow" disease outbreak that in turn led to cases of acute-onset Creutzfeldt-Jakob disease (CJD) in people resulted from the transfer of a similar prion.

The idea that is most favored for the crossover of HIV strains into our species is that these viruses "jumped" during the harvesting of "bush meat." As human population sizes have increased and starvation has become an ever-present threat, the practice of killing wild-living primates (bush meat) for human food is thought to have become much more prevalent. An obvious possibility is that someone could have cut their hand and contracted one or other HIV variant as a consequence of blood contaminating an open wound while butchering a chimp, a gorilla or a sooty mangabey. Once that happened, all the epidemiological data we have is consistent with the perception that sexual transmission has been, and is, the main mechanism of HIV spread. Some aggressive attempts have been made to suggest that HIV was widely disseminated via "early" (before we knew anything about HIV/AIDS) vaccines and immunization campaigns but, following careful, retrospective analysis, no evidence has been found to support this view.

Was AIDS active much earlier in Africa?

Probably, but not in a big way: even with the possibility that some cases were missed because they were thought of as bacterial infections, a cause that could be eliminated by antibiotic treatment from the time that such drugs became available, the disease incidence could only have been a minute fraction of the current situation. That doesn't exclude the possibility that there may have been occasional outbreaks of AIDS in remote regions long before it came to the attention of the international medical and scientific community. When, for example, we review the situation for the influenza pandemic of 1918–1919, there aren't good mortality records for many isolated communities that were governed by one or other European colonial power.

Given that AIDS presents clinically as a wasting disease, with death ultimately resulting from some other infection, a chronic HIV problem in a remote African village, for instance, could have gone largely unnoticed or been attributed to some other pathogen or malnutrition. The underlying cause could easily be missed. It was not until the 1970s that scientists like Robert Gallo of the U.S. National Cancer Institute developed the lymphocyte culture techniques that enabled the initial isolation of HIV.

As it is, there are likely African AIDS cases from 1958–1959, and we know (by recovering HIV from stored tissues) of an African American teenager, Robert R., who died from this infection in 1969. Also, it is definitively established that throughout the 1970s several Europeans succumbed to AIDS. According to the later molecular archaeology analysis of HIV-1 sequences, the virus became established in humans sometime between 1915 and 1941, likely in the 1930s. This was a pandemic that was waiting to happen. The expansion of African road systems, the greater numbers of sexually active and promiscuous long-distance truck drivers, and the massive increase in international air travel all contributed to the global spread of HIV.

Does the immune system fail totally when confronted with HIV?

That's the final outcome and, by definition, AIDS and immune failure are synonymous. But AIDS doesn't develop immediately. The immune system works well initially in people infected with HIV, and even untreated (with drugs), they can remain relatively well for a year or longer in some cases. However, there is a constant, ongoing, battle in the "deep background" of the apparently healthy individual's lymph nodes and spleen as HIV-specific CD8+ killer T lymphocytes function to eliminate the infected CD4+ helper T cells. That war is fought strictly on the lines of Darwinian evolution (favoring the rapidly replicating virus), and is inevitably lost as mutants emerge and immune-escape from CD8+ T cell-mediated control leads irrevocably to the depletion of the CD4+ population. Once these helpers that maintain the overall integrity of the immune system are destroyed, the CD8+ killers soon become "exhausted," ineffectual, and, toward the end, disappear.

Death from AIDS is generally caused by uncontrolled infection with organisms like TB (*M. tuberculosis*) or other atypical mycobacteria like *M. avium* that are normally dealt with by CD4+ and CD8+ T cells. Well-controlled commensals, like the fungus *Pneumocystis carinii* and the protozoan *Cryptosporidium jiroveci* (formerly *C. parvum*), that live relatively amiably on the mucosal surfaces in the respiratory tract and gut of healthy adults can also invade and cause lethal disease. Then, though less commonly, the final blow may be delivered by the cancer-causing gammaherpesviruses, Epstein Barr virus (EBV) and Kaposi's sarcoma virus (KSHV). Other persistent human herpesviruses (HHVs) that manifest normally as transient infections of childhood (HHV6 and 7) can also reactivate and cause severe problems in AIDS patients. The same is true for cytomegalovirus (CMV or HHV5).

Medical science was unaware of KSHV and HHV6 before the beginning of the HIV pandemic. Prior to AIDS, the characteristic, purplish/black Kaposi's sarcoma was a rare skin tumor seen in elderly men of Mediterranean origin and, more commonly, in young people from parts of Sub-Saharan Africa. Kaposi's was "outed" as a virus-induced cancer by HIV, though we already knew about EBV, which causes infectious mononucleosis in adolescents and, for most of us, persists as a generally unapparent infection throughout long lives. In Western societies, EBV is known to induce relatively rare lymphomas that emerge after, say, the treatment of cancer patients with radiation and highly toxic drugs that compromise the immune system and, consequently, EBV control.

Chronic malaria infection is also linked to the EBV-associated Burkitt's lymphoma, a visually dreadful tumor of the head and neck that afflicts young people in some developing countries. Like AIDS, malaria is broadly immunosuppressive, though not as a consequence of the precise targeting of CD4+ T cells. Burkitt's lymphoma is 1,000 times more common in AIDS patients. That cancer/AIDS correlation is not, however, obvious for another EBV-associated tumor, the nasopharyngeal carcinoma (NPC) that is particularly prevalent in southern China. What this suggests is that the part played by CD8+ and, perhaps, by CD4+ killer T cells in limiting the emergence of Burkitt's lymphoma and Kaposi's sarcoma is less important when it comes to NPC.

How does HIV target the CD4+ T cell?

As discussed earlier, viruses only grow within living cells where, like a "cuckoo in the nest," they exploit elements of the normal molecular machinery. The virion (virus particle) thus needs some mechanism for gaining access to the cell cytoplasm and/or nucleus. It just so happens that HIV binds directly and very specifically to both the CD4 molecule and to another protein, the chemokine receptor type 5 (CCR5), both of which are found on the surface of helper T lymphocytes. That insight emerged when it was realized that a small number of individuals with a mutation that results in the failure to express CCR5 did not contract the most commonly transmissible form of HIV-1, despite pursuing lifestyles that left them very exposed to the virus.

Do we yet have a vaccine for AIDS?

Despite spending, in one estimate, more than $650 million dollars annually on trying to develop an AIDS vaccine, we do not yet have an effective product. Some progress has been made, and a recent trial showed around 20–30% protection, but there's obviously a way to go. That sounds like not all that much for a whole lot of money, but the yearly investment is less than the cost of replacing one B2 stealth bomber: the first 20 such aircraft came in at $2.2 billion each.

Along the way we've learned a very great deal about how the human immune system works, but the problem is that, once in the body, HIV changes constantly, throwing off mutants that both escape immune control and are able to infect other people. A single individual can end up with multiple HIV variants circulating concurrently in the blood. This propensity for change, along with the fact that HIV persists and cannot be fully eliminated by either immune response mechanisms or by drug treatment, makes the development of an effective vaccine extraordinarily difficult.

Still, we need to keep trying. An unknown virus that is just as difficult to deal with after gaining access to the human body, but much more infectious than HIV, could be out there in some wildlife reservoir. We can't give up on the effort to make an AIDS vaccine. Also, as discussed below, other public and private funds allocated to AIDS research have paid off with the development of very effective drugs.

Will we ever have a vaccine for AIDS?

The simple answer is: we don't know, though there has been limited progress recently. What we do understand, though, is that pursuing the types of relatively simple strategies that have led to effective vaccines that protect against many other viruses just doesn't work when we are trying to counter highly variable pathogens, like HIV and hepatitis C virus, that establish persistent infections and change within us. Currently, perhaps the most interesting possibility is that we might be able to make an "end run" around HIV variability by figuring out how to "trick" the immune system into recognizing conserved, invariant parts of the virus that can't be changed (mutate) without compromising viral "fitness" (capacity to invade and to multiply).

We know that there are rare, naturally occurring antibodies that do bind to conserved regions of HIV, but we've yet to develop a product that, when injected, can induce such responses. At the moment, this approach seems to be one of the most promising areas of inquiry.

I already mentioned the recent multipartner Thai trial RV144 (involving the U.S. military, NIH, Thai Ministry of Health, Sanofi/Pasteur, Genentech, and Vaxgen) of a prime/boost AIDS vaccine strategy that surprised and delighted AIDS researchers when it gave what has variously been interpreted as a 24–33% level of protection. Clearly, even if this holds up on further analysis, there is a very long way to go before anything could be made available commercially, but it does suggest that progress is possible.

Has science failed us when it comes to HIV/AIDS?

No, absolutely not: as in the case of SARS, science has done a great job with this extraordinarily difficult infection. When AIDS first hit in a big way in 1981, most who contracted the disease were dead within 18–24 months. If that had happened 30 years earlier, we would not have had the technology to deal with it, or even to make a good diagnosis. Now, those who have access to therapy live relatively normal life spans. Back in 1981, when physicians in San Francisco, New York, and Europe first identified this new, progressive, wasting condition, the essentially symptomatic diagnosis gave rise to acronyms like GRID (gay-related immunodeficiency disease). Many speculated that it was a consequence of lifestyle choices, including the use of "recreational" drugs. There was no consensus that GRID was infectious. The gay community became very defensive, while elements of the "moral majority" were satisfied with the conclusion that this was some type of divine punishment. Given these perceptions, think of what might have happened socially if the situation had persisted and this mysterious disease continued to spread. As it was, both attitudes had long-term consequences, with the gays reacting too slowly when the true cause was determined and reactionary politicians blocking open discussion and obvious protective measures (like needle exchange) to limit HIV spread.

The beginnings of a rational policy approach to limit the incidence of AIDS, as the disease was soon more commonly known, came in 1983, when Pasteur Institute scientists Françoise Barré-Sinoussi and Luc Montagnier isolated the causative virus. This in turn led quickly (from 1985) to the broad availability of a specific diagnostic test. Even with that assay in place and clear evidence that AIDS is a virus-induced disease, there was still in some quarters considerable opposition to testing the blood supply. The resultant delay led to many being infected with contaminated blood and blood products, both in Europe and the United States. Now, blood transfusion is generally safe, and new assays ensure that even the most minimal risk of contamination can be detected prior to use.

In time, epidemiologists would have shown that the disease is indeed transmitted by infected blood, but the fact that the onset of AIDS can be slow could have confounded the analysis and confused the situation for years, especially when there were economic pressures that worked against efforts to secure the blood supply. Knowing that the virus is in the circulation system further provided insight into the nature of sexual transmission. It became obvious that this disease is by no means restricted to men who have sex with men—a reality that emerged later in Africa and Southeast Asia, where AIDS is predominantly a heterosexual disease. Men and women who take sensible precautions are unlikely to become infected, but that insight comes only with understanding.

What progress has been made in the last 25 years?

A great deal: while the immunologists haven't yet been able to develop a protective vaccine, the chemists working in both government-funded research laboratories and the pharmaceutical industry have been remarkably successful. As mentioned earlier, HIV-infected individuals live essentially normal lives if they have access to HAART (highly active anti-retroviral therapy). In the wealthier countries, that means treatment with at least three drugs that target different aspects of the virus replication cycle.

The first drug approved for the treatment of HIV was the nuceloside/nucleotide RT inhibitor *Ziduvidine* in 1987. Others, like the non-nucleotide RT inhibitor *Nevirapine* (1996), followed. By 1995, infectious disease physicians also had the first of the protease inhibitors, *Saquinavir*, that target enzymes required for the assembly of new virus particles. Then there are the integrase inhibitors and the maturation inhibitors that hit other points in the virus life cycle. The consequence is that individuals persistently infected with HIV now take a cocktail of drugs (HAART) that operate via a variety of mechanisms to prevent virus replication. As we have understood for decades with cancer therapy, hitting a number of different molecular targets simultaneously prevents the emergence of drug-resistant escape mutants.

Apart from the fact that most people on HAART have reasonable life spans, taking these drugs means that there is only minimal, if any, HIV in the blood and, as a consequence, a greatly diminished risk of sexual transmission. In addition, circumcision has been shown to confer a considerable measure of protection for heterosexuals, though that is less clear for men who have sex with men. Trials are also in progress with drug-containing gels that, when used topically prior to coition, may contribute to limiting the incidence of infection in women. Even for those in poor countries who are not receiving HAART, the risk of mother-to-child transmission, which happens at birth (via blood) or after (via milk), may also be substantially decreased. An anti-retrovirus drug is given from 28 weeks of pregnancy, then (to both mother and child) for at least a week thereafter. Similarly, post-exposure HAART following something like an accidental "stick" with an HIV-contaminated needle has shown a good level of success.

The situation is constantly improving, though a slight upturn in infection rates among at-risk individuals in some advanced countries emphasizes the fact that it is important to persist with education (particularly for those who have never seen the horror of frank AIDS), safe sex practices, and generally responsible and open behavior. As anyone who has tried to stay with a strict diet knows, when things are going well it's very easy for us to let down our guard and relax our standards. Being a bit overweight is one thing, but who would want to be infected with this horrible virus and, as a consequence, have to confess the fact to possible sex partners while taking masses of pills each day?

Could AIDS blow up in some way to cause an even bigger problem?

New variants of the AIDS virus emerge constantly, and it is now well established that people can be infected from the outset with more than one strain. In addition, there is evidence that super-infection with novel HIV strains can occur in those who are already HIV positive. Despite that, even if a totally new sexually transmitted human retrovirus came onto the scene, there's no particular reason to think that it would cause more difficulties than the HIV types that are currently circulating. The great majority of the human family remain uninfected. Most are safe because they do not inject drugs, are celibate, or are in stable sexual relationships with trusted partners. For those who will take risks, it seems that downing an anti-retroviral drug prior to sexual activity may provide a good measure of protection. So long as those behavior patterns persist, our species is in no danger of being wiped out by this disease.

The only thing that gives a sense of vague (and probably unwarranted) concern is that the virus might suddenly change in a way that permits a different form of spread. If, for example, an HIV variant emerged that, like influenza or TB, could infect readily via the respiratory route, we could all be in real trouble. An absolute horror scenario for any medical epidemiologist or infectious disease physician is an airborne virus that initially causes an essentially mild, or even unapparent, infection, and then develops later into an inexorably fatal disease. A distantly related retrovirus that causes a lung adenocarcinoma (Jaagsiekte) of sheep may transmit (though poorly) via the respiratory route. Any such switch is highly improbable for HIV. Still, there can be no absolute certainties when it comes to virus variation. Experimental biologists like me are well aware of Murphy's Law: "Anything that can go wrong will go wrong."

What might cause HIV to change in some dramatic and unpredictable way? My main concern is that, with extensive drug treatment, we are subjecting this virus to enormous selective pressure. That's not so much of an issue with those who are maintaining a strict HAART regime. As discussed above, having three drugs in a mix that targets different pathways makes the emergence of resistant mutants extremely unlikely.

Apart from possible interruptions to supply, the problem in some developing countries is that, while lifesaving anti-HIV drugs are indeed being distributed, those who are being treated will likely receive only a single product. Additionally, there often isn't the medical infrastructure in place to ensure adequate follow-up or advice on appropriate use. Not taking the drugs routinely, or splitting the pills to share with others, can lead to treatment "holidays" that favor the emergence of viral mutants. There's no reason that any such mutation should lead to a virus with a modified transmission profile, but this is one area where any unmonitored change is potentially dangerous.

Once in the human body, can HIV ever be eliminated?

Perhaps at some time in the future this will be possible, though the development of any safe, practicable way for curing established HIV infections in large numbers of people looks to be very remote at the moment. Even so, molecular science is moving with enormous speed. Advances in our understanding over the past decades have led to the identification of a spectrum of genetic strategies for limiting, or preventing, HIV infection in laboratory-cultured CD4+ T cells. Prominent among these inhibitors are the small interfering (si) RNAs, which belong to a family of regulatory molecules that interfere with specific genes in various ways to prevent viral protein production. The discovery of these regulatory RNAs earned Andrew Fox and Craig Mello the 2006 Nobel Prize for Medicine.

The entry of HIV into the T lymphocyte can, for example, be substantially blocked by pre-treating with an siRNA that prevents the expression of the CCR5 receptor molecule (see above). Of course, that would be of no value if the cell is already infected, but there are other siRNAs that can limit virus replication by perturbing various molecular pathways. Applying that type of technology is fine if we're talking about CD4+ T cells that have been taken from the blood of an infected person for treatment in the laboratory, but the problem is to get such products to the right place when they are simply injected into the patient's arm. Achieving such "targeted" delivery is an issue for any form of selective therapy.

That difficulty is often solved by the use of small, synthetic molecules (drugs) that go most places in the body. Even then, while most of the HAART drugs do not cross the tight junctions of the blood-brain barrier, the severity of HIV-related neurological problems is greatly diminished in treated HIV carriers. That could reflect that, while activated T lymphocytes and macrophages are known to transit into normal brain from the blood, HAART treatment will mean that there are no freshly infected cells to make this journey.

One "cure" strategy that has been tested is to take normal T cells from HAART-treated individuals, incubate with siRNAs or other molecular inhibitors of HIV infection/replication, and then infuse these "protected" lymphocytes back into the patient. Repeating this process a number of times leads to a progressive buildup in the numbers of resistant T cells and the possibility that, at least for a time, drug treatment can be withdrawn. As things stand, of course, that is an experimental rather than a practical strategy for limiting HIV infection, probably in the relatively short term.

Some AIDS patients who later developed lymphomas have been treated with massive doses of cytotoxic drugs and irradiation to eliminate the tumor. This process also destroys the bone marrow (BM) populations that are the progenitors of the red and white blood cells, including the CD4+ and CD8+ T lymphocytes. As a consequence, the immune system has to be reconstituted by the infusion of BM from a matched (for transplantation type) uninfected individual. That provides the opportunity to treat the entire BM population, including the CD4+ T lymphocyte precursors, with a cocktail of siRNAs and other molecules designed to block HIV infection and/or replication.

Then, a patient given BM from a naturally HIV-resistant CCR5- donor effectively controlled the infection because the target CCR5-CD4+ T cells that developed over the subsequent months from the BM graft were no longer susceptible to infection. That raises the long-term possibility of using gene therapy approaches to take a "homologous" BM sample from an infected individual, and then knock out (disrupt) the CCR5 gene, prior to expanding these cells in culture and infusing them back into the patient. This kind of experiment is done all the time in lab mice, but there's "many a slip twixt cup and lip" when it comes to scaling up any technology from short-lived rodents to humans.

The limited results to date look promising, but BM ablation and reconstitution is an extraordinarily expensive and dangerous procedure that could only ever be applied to very few patients. Still, if we could go down the homologous BM/ gene therapy mode (using the patient's own BM), it may not be necessary to first compromise the immune system if simply infusing HIV-resistant cells leads to the gradual replacement of the susceptible set. At present, so long as HAART therapy works and there is no superimposed cancer problem, this is not a realistic option. But there is reason to think that targeted molecular blocking strategies may someday be practicable for limiting the growth of HIV in patients.

The Bottom Line

Most of us are at no risk for HIV/AIDS if we don't inject drugs and are celibate, or continue to practice safe sex. The only nightmare scenario is having a serious accident in a country where the blood supply is not secure. The emergence of some new AIDS virus is not a particular concern, unless a novel variant changes its mode of transmission, a very unlikely possibility. Those who are infected survive on HAART therapy, but the much better option is to take reasonable care and avoid being exposed in the first place. At this stage, there's no obvious vaccine strategy that is likely to work, at least in the near term. There are other treatment possibilities including, for example, various forms of gene therapy, but these have not developed to the stage where they are practicable for even very limited use.

9

MAD COWS AND
CREUTZFELDT-JAKOB DISEASE

*Has there ever been a mad cow or Creutzfeldt-Jakob
disease pandemic?*

No, but it is worth reminding ourselves of these "scary
monsters" as we think about novel pandemic threats. What
we're discussing here is the link between bovine spongiform
encephalopathy (BSE), or mad cow disease, and the somewhat
similar human condition, variant Creutzfeldt-Jakob disease
(vCJD). This particular combination caused major concerns
in the medical and veterinary infectious disease communities
through the last decades of the twentieth century. While isolated cases of vCJD were recorded in many countries (including Japan, the United States, and Canada), the epicenter was in
the United Kingdom and Europe. The disease did manifest in
different regions of the world, but the experience could hardly
be called a pandemic. Despite early fears, there was no evidence of horizontal or vertical transmission between humans,
and the numbers of people affected proved ultimately to be
quite low.

Anything that compromises the food supply is, though, of
enormous public concern. The thought that we could contract
an inexorably progressive, fatal neurological condition simply by going out for a steak or roast beef dinner, especially

when we're on an international vacation, struck at the core of what most regard as a basic right for traveling omnivores. The BSE/vCJD story rang some loud alarm bells, both about the nature of human food production and the possibility that unconventional infectious agents could constitute an increasing risk factor.

So what is spongiform encephalopathy?

The term comes from the neuropathologists, the people who conduct postmortems and then look down optical microscopes to examine very thin, stained slices of the brain and spinal cord. What they could see in brains that had first been preserved in formalin and then embedded in hot paraffin wax prior to cutting (sectioning) with the ultra-sharp blade of a microtome—like a lab guillotine that shaves a surface rather than amputates—was a brain shot through with holes. There looked to be circumscribed holes in the cytoplasm of the nerve cells themselves, and spaces with no discernible substance or structure in the surrounding tissue (or neuropil). The brain sections thus had an abnormal sponge-like appearance, a spongiform encephalopathy or, less respectfully in the specialist community, a "spongy brain-rot." This is, to state the obvious, not something you want happening inside your head. Even worse, nobody likes to think that such a condition could be "out there" in some infectious form. The greatest fear for many of us is loss of intellectual competence and brain function, and we don't like to think that it is catching.

The transmissible spongiform encephalopathies (TSEs) comprise a frightening family of infections that were, until comparatively recently, quite mysterious. The prototype is scrapie, the chronic, progressive, and ultimately fatal disease of sheep. Long known to be a problem in (particularly) parts of Scandinavia and Scotland, scrapie is named for the fact that afflicted animals develop a severe pruritis (itching) and rub their wool off by "scraping" against a fence post or some other solid object. The itching sensation results from the very characteristic, spongy brain damage and, since the 1930s, it has been known that this disease spreads horizontally within sheep and goat populations. Whether or not vertical transmission occurs prior to birth is less clear, with there being minimal evidence that it may pass from ewe to lamb. Cows, mice and hamsters ultimately develop both the characteristic neurological symptoms and pathology following the injection of filtered (to remove bacteria), ground-up material directly into the brain, but scrapie has not been shown to cause any naturally occurring disease in cattle, or to be a problem for meat eaters like dogs and humans.

If the TSEs are infections, what's the big mystery?

The fascination of scientists with scrapie stemmed from the fact that, despite many years of very sustained effort and the fact that the disease was long known to be transmissible by needle to other sheep and to some rodents, the researchers were unable either to isolate a causative virus or to show that the fluid supernates from ground-up, infected tissues containing detectable nucleic acids (RNA or DNA). The scrapie agent, whatever it was, passed through filters with very small pores that would hold back any known pathogen. Furthermore, unlike all RNA and DNA viruses, it survived both heating to high temperatures (including exposure to boiling water for several hours) and treatment with toxic chemicals like formalin (formaldehyde).

Then, over the ensuing decades, scientists including Vincent Zigas, John Mathews, Michael Alpers, Joe Gibbs, and Carleton Gadjusek (Nobel Prize 1976) worked out that a similar spongiform encephalopathy, the fatal paralysis known as kuru, was being maintained in the Fore people of Papua New Guinea by their practice of ritual cannibalism. Furthermore, as with scrapie in sheep and goats, kuru could be transmitted by injecting clarified, human brain material into non-human primates. On top of that, the pathologically identical human condition, Creutzfeldt-Jakob disease (CJD), was inadvertently transmitted to others by the transplantation of corneas from people who had died with severe dementia, and via formalin-treated stereotactic needles (inserted in the brain for locating structures during neurosurgery) that had been used previously on a CJD patient. Collectively, along with a comparable disease of mink that was initially thought to have originated from these small carnivores being fed scrapie-infected sheep offal, these conditions became known collectively as the TSEs.

Despite the fact that the TSEs could be induced in other species following injection, we were not particularly concerned that these diseases would transfer from animals to man. After all, it was abundantly clear that, for centuries, human beings had been eating mutton, roast lamb, sheep shanks, sheep stomachs (haggis), and even brains from animals that must have been incubating scrapie. Then, from 1995, cases of rapid-onset "variant" CJD (vCJD) began to emerge in the United Kingdom in 16- to 30-year-olds. Prior to that, CJD was considered to be a slow, progressive condition affecting older people. The connection to mad cow disease, BSE, was immediate.

First diagnosed by British veterinary neuropathologists in 1986, the nine-year interval between the recognition of BSE and the onset of vCJD in humans was in accord with what we knew about the TSEs. More than 60 years of studying scrapie experimentally had told us that the incubation period in sheep can be very long indeed. Given the high beef consumption by British residents and tourists, the immediate possibility was that we could be facing a slowly emerging, global tragedy involving hundreds of thousands, if not millions, of people. Fortunately, the numbers of those afflicted has been in the hundreds and, with the control of BSE, the problem seems to have gone away.

Did BSE originate from sheep scrapie?

That's one possibility. The source of infection for cattle is thought to have been animal products, particularly bone meal. With more than 7 billion people who need to eat each day, any source of high value protein is valuable and, if available in large quantities, can ultimately influence (or contaminate) what emerges at the top of the food chain. Abattoir waste, including blood, bones, and so forth, is subject to heat treatment (called rendering) prior to being ground up for use in animal feed. A British decision to drop the maximum temperature required for the rendering process is thought to have allowed the survival of the BSE agent. Could that have come originally from infected sheep tissues? Perhaps, but recent genetic analysis suggests that the disease may have arisen from a spontaneous mutation in cattle. How would that work?

Over the past decades, neuropathologists and neurochemists have concluded that many dementias are caused by the accumulation of mis-folded, non-functional proteins in the brain, to give substances like the amyloid characteristic of Alzheimer's disease. Though Alzheimer's disease is not known to be infectious, the TSEs are broadly similar pathologically and are thought to reflect somewhat comparable processes. The 1997 Nobel Prize for Physiology or Medicine was awarded to California medical scientist Stanley Prusiner for his discovery that diseases like scrapie, vCJD, kuru, and BSE are caused by an abnormal protein, the prion (PrP). As a protein rather than nucleic acid, the PrP is very resistant to heat and to chemical degradation. When transferred to a previously uninfected individual, TSE prions serve as a template for the inappropriate folding of otherwise normal self-proteins, which can in turn both cause and further transmit the disease.

What now seems likely is that the TSEs of different species can develop spontaneously as a consequence of chance mutations in the gene that encodes the "healthy" form of the PrP. The frightening thing about that idea is that it could occur anywhere at any time. How did humans contract the vCJD TSE from cattle? In the absence of very careful trimming, beef cuts are likely to contain nerve fibers and other elements of neural tissue. That's the probable source of the abnormal bovine PrP that infected the 166 Britons and 44 others who developed vCJD as a consequence of eating meat from animals that were incubating BSE.

At least for a time, the roast beef of England got a very bad name. The lack of scrapie transmission to people may simply reflect that the variant sheep PrP is simply too unlike the normal human PrP form to induce any abnormal folding. The BSE PrP also caused disease in zoo animals, namely big cats and non-human primates that were fed contaminated beef, and it is thought that some outbreaks of mink encephalopathy resulted from the same cause. Most of the cattle that developed BSE in the United Kingdom were probably infected as a consequence of eating inadequately rendered bone meal and the like, with there being little evidence of horizontal transmission between animals. The disease also went international as a consequence of exporting both bone meal and British cattle to other countries, including Canada. The lesson here is, of course, that it can be dangerous to feed animal products to any species that is used for human consumption. At a minimum, such material should be heated to very high temperatures.

What is "bone meal"?

Used as fertilizer, crushed and coarsely ground bones provide a good source of phosphorous and calcium to promote plant growth. For the same reason crushed bone meal has also been fed to cattle and other livestock.

Has anyone contracted vCJD from eating imported British beef?

There were, perhaps, two cases in Saudi Arabia, but the proven instances of vCJD in foreign nationals who ate British beef were in tourists who visited the United Kingdom before the BSE/vCJD link became obvious. Infected cattle were also exported to a number of European and a few Asian countries. France, for example, banned British beef and cattle imports from 1996 to 2002. The beef industries in both Canada and the United States were also damaged, with the suspected origin of at least some North American BSE cases being "rendered" material from an English cow imported to Canada. In all, more than 190,000 cattle are thought to have contracted BSE worldwide, with 183,000+ of those cases being in Britain. Some 3 million UK cattle were slaughtered; the cost of the epidemic reached £720 million a year, and estimates of the ultimate economic loss are as high as £39 billion.

Was there even the possibility of a BSE/vCJD pandemic?

That could, perhaps, have happened 200 years ago, but we were saved by modern science. As with many infectious disease problems, our ultimate protection was that careful investigative studies by epidemiologists, pathologists, and others, together with the earlier discovery of prions by Stan Prusiner, allowed us to understand what was happening. As a consequence, the regulatory authorities were able to take appropriate preventive steps. Fortunately, the incidence of oral transmission to humans must have been very low. Clearly, the BSE PrP transmitted much more readily to cattle.

Different PrPs are found in many species (including fungi), and it is intriguing that only the bovine (or human) variants are, to date, of direct concern to us. As things stand, in the absence of solid evidence for vertical transmission, the likelihood of becoming infected with a human PrP is currently minimal.

Does the history of BSE/CJD raise other concerns?

Yes: North American cervids (mule deer, white tailed deer, elk, and moose) are known to develop a TSE-associated chronic wasting disease, with evidence of the problem now recorded in 12 U.S. states and two Canadian provinces. This cervid TSE has been shown to transmit horizontally following the ingestion of PrPs excreted onto pasture, but there is no evidence to date that the disease can cross over into cattle, sheep, or humans. Even so, a future mutational change in a gene coding for a normal human (or animal) PrP may lead to the production of protein that is much more infectious for us. Also, though nobody seems to have looked seriously at the possibility that North American squirrels develop a TSE-like disease, limited clinical findings from Kentucky/Appalachia suggest that both CJD and Parkinson's disease may be associated with a local practice of eating squirrel brains.

Are the TSEs a pandemic risk?

The likelihood of such a pandemic is very remote, but not completely impossible: in general, the lack of any evidence for the environmental (as distinct from surgical) transmission of CJD and the low incidence of human vCJD in those who were potentially exposed to BSE-contaminated beef indicates that these PrPs are not particularly infectious. Even so, any transmissible condition that is silent for years prior to manifesting as an inexorably progressive, ultimately fatal disease does raise a very big red flag. The concern is that, if something novel of this type emerged that was highly infectious, it could spread globally before we even recognized the problem. It's stretching a very long bow, but think what could happen if a PrP-like protein were to be present in milk and survive the manufacturing process for making those fine cheeses and exotic chocolates that are exported around the planet.

The warning that the BSE experience sounds is also that, as we move forward with the extraordinary technologies that we are now beginning to control, we should exercise great care with any product that is designed to be both very small and self-replicating. I would not want to suggest for one moment that we should delay the development of, for example, micro-machines or therapeutic approaches based in molecular and/or nanotechnology, but it would be prudent to require rigorous safety testing. I know that some are concerned about genetically modified organisms for similar reasons but, though I believe that safety testing is important, the fact that the genes used to generate drought-resistant plants and so forth are distributed broadly through biology and the foodstuffs that humans (and other species) normally eat gives me much less cause for concern.

10

ECONOMICS AND THE HUMAN-ANIMAL EQUATION

What type of pandemic infection causes the most economic damage?

The SARS experience taught us that a mysterious, rapidly spreading, and potentially fatal respiratory infection can trigger a short, sharp, severe economic shock that has longer term consequences. Though less than 900 people died from SARS and Toronto was the only city hit outside the Asia Pacific region, the losses to airlines, the hospitality sector, and all those associated with the travel industry were estimated at around $50 billion. Two years later, the big hotels in Singapore and Toronto were still recovering. Contrast that with the situation for seasonal influenza: the calculated mortality based on "excess deaths" in the United States alone ranges from 20,000 to 40,000 (250,000–500,000 worldwide) for any given flu year. But influenza is familiar, many of us will have been vaccinated, and the fact that one of the standard strains is circulating does not cause business travelers and tourists to stop flying or induce most people outside Asia to wear face masks in the streets and in airports.

Even so, the CDC economists estimate that the total US economic burden, including loss of productivity, hospitalization, and so forth, is in excess of $80 billion for a "normal" influenza year. It may be too soon to cost the "mild" 2009 SW

H1N1 pandemic, though a 2006 economic modeling exercise put the global expense of an influenza pandemic in the $330 billion to $4.4 trillion range, depending on the severity of the disease. Of course, as the global financial crisis of 2007 taught us, the economic damage that can be done by New York bankers and financial speculators operating in a poorly conceived and administered regulatory framework can be much greater, but the cost of a global infectious disease pandemic is still very substantial, in addition to the enormous social dislocation.

Is a novel respiratory infection the only economic threat?

No, but the point about respiratory viruses is that they can be hard, if not impossible, to contain. Once diagnosed, it is a somewhat more straightforward matter to isolate people with a newly emerged, severe GI tract infection that presents with characteristic symptoms of diarrhea and/or vomiting. That's much more difficult, though, when large numbers of people are confined to, say, a school, a hospital, or a cruise ship. Also, unless we are seeing the reemergence of cholera or typhoid in one of the advanced countries, most outbreaks of gastro-enteritis (induced by a spectrum of virus, bacterial, and even parasitic infections) will, like many "colds" and "flu-like" conditions, generally be accepted as part of the "normal disease background" and will not trigger any drastic action.

That doesn't mean that there is no significant financial burden. A 1995 study suggested that rotavirus induced diarrhea in 5- to 8-year-olds was responsible for $564 million in medical expenses alone in the United States, a draw-down on the economy that has hopefully been mitigated by the subsequent introduction of an effective vaccine. There is as yet no commercial vaccine to protect against the noroviruses. But, with a CDC figure of some 21 million cases annually and a likely 2–4 days of illness, the loss in productivity must be considerable. One analysis of a 2003 outbreak in a UK hospital calculated the damage at around £280,000, a substantial figure in any constrained health care budget. Similarly, if we think in terms of familiar, endemic respiratory infections, the common cold has been estimated to cost the United States $40 billion annually in medical treatment, work absences (particularly young parents), and generally diminished productivity.

At least in societies that have good medical and public health coverage, the sudden appearance of very characteristic infections that are spread by insect vectors (dengue, yellow fever) can easily be managed to minimize the risk of further transmission. Even so, the costs can be substantial. After the initial 1999 incursion in New York City, West Nile virus traveled slowly across the United States using a mosquito/bird and occasional mammal (horse/human) life cycle. Analyzing the consequences of the 2005 Sacramento outbreak (169 human cases), Robert Peterson and colleagues estimated the financial damage at about $3 million. That would have been replicated in many cities across North America as the virus spread North and South, and from the East to the West.

Will it be massively expensive if quarantine officials are suddenly faced with an emergency?

It depends on whether the problem is caught at point of entry. A likely scenario is that an individual on an incoming international flight develops symptoms of some severe, exotic infectious disease, perhaps one of the viral hemorrhagic fevers. Most acute virus infections have an incubation period (to first clinical signs) of less than 7 days, so the quarantine authorities might require that the other passengers be held for two weeks for continued observation. The old coastal or island quarantine stations that were used to isolate sick immigrants arriving on passenger ships have all been closed, so how would this be done? One strategy is to turn a vacant airport hangar into a temporary quarantine facility. Hangars are generally isolated in a sea of tarmac, so they provide a good level of separation, and cities served by major international airports are likely to have contractors who can supply chemical toilets, shower trailers, and other necessities at short notice. Providing there is no secondary spread, the total cost to an airport of confining, say, 200 people for two weeks under these conditions has been estimated at around $300,000. Then there would be other expenses associated with the attendance of medical personnel, laboratory testing, and so forth.

The expense could be infinitely greater if the affected patient is not diagnosed until later, the other passengers on the flight have to be located and (perhaps) recalled, and there is the possibility of further contact in the community. Still, imported (and generally mild) cases of SARS were identified in more than 30 countries, but few people were affected, and there was no incidence of secondary spread and little direct economic consequence. Canada seems to have been unfortunate in that the individual who brought SARS to Toronto was highly infectious. In fact, the SARS experience emphasizes how chance can determine the consequences of any disease incursion, at least for most pathogens. Influenza, on the other hand, teaches us a different lesson. Once a novel and highly infectious influenza strain is established in any human community, no matter how small, there is a reasonable possibility that it will go around the world.

From a financial standpoint, does influenza remain our main concern?

Influenza is probably the biggest financial concern when we talk only of known human diseases, but there is another scenario in which massive economic damage can result—when a known infection is diagnosed in a country that was thought to be free and clear. What we're talking about here is some identifiable condition affecting domestic animals in, for example, a nation that derives substantial income from animal-based agriculture. And it doesn't need to be a zoonosis, an infection that transmits from animals to people. A pandemic that affects large numbers of economically important livestock can be a national disaster.

Foot and mouth disease (FMD), for example, is caused by a highly infectious picornavirus (from the same family as polio) that transmits to most cloven-hoofed ruminants (cattle, pigs, sheep, goats, deer). Totally unrelated to the hand, foot, and mouth disease that affects small children, there have been rare cases of people contracting FMD (though none since 1966), and it does not spread to humans as a consequence of eating infected meat. Mainly a problem for commercial cattle, sheep, and pig production, FMD virus causes fever, the ulceration of mucus membranes, and productivity loss in cattle, rather than a high incidence of mortality. There are a number of different FMD strains and, unlike the situation for the related human poliovirus, the available vaccines are not particularly effective at inducing long-term protective immunity.

Why is FMD so damaging?

Infected animals can be culled rapidly, so it might seem that FMD wouldn't have a lasting impact. However, these viruses are extremely hardy and are easily spread by contaminated boots, automobile tires, and the like. As a consequence, entire areas have to be effectively quarantined. In the British 2001 epidemic, for example, the Isle of Man Grand Prix was canceled, leading to considerable economic loss for local businesses, especially hotels and restaurants. I was working in a veterinary research institute in Edinburgh during the 1967 UK FMD outbreak. There was a sign on the gate, stating: "no entry for vehicles from England," and that wasn't just a reflection of the Scottish nationalist sentiments that were being expressed rather aggressively at that distant time.

The 2001 UK FMD outbreak resulted in the culling of 10 million sheep, cattle, and pigs, with a calculated £8 billion total cost to the British economy. A substantial component was lost tourist income. A separate estimate that looked only at the situation for Scotland came up with a figure of £250 million. And the British Isles are small in total land area, with both cattle and sheep agriculture being closely monitored. Where FMD has historically been even more devastating is in large countries like Argentina, where herds are scattered and beef/ livestock exports are of substantial economic importance. All nations are vulnerable, with Korea, Japan, and Bulgaria seeing outbreaks in 2010–2011.

Then, apart from the financial, social, and emotional costs associated with killing and burying (or burning) infected livestock and "in contact" flocks and herds, the cessation of exports from affected nations that were previously free of the disease inevitably has a major economic impact. Inability to supply can lead to the transient, or even permanent, loss of markets, with trade only being resumed when the country in question is ultimately declared to be disease free. In short, the problem with a veterinary epidemic can be as much the international regulatory and quarantine requirements that are designed to limit the global spread of infection as the extent and duration of the disease outbreak. Local producers in the importing countries may also have a vested financial interest in applying political pressure to delay the resumption of trade for as long as possible.

Could there ever be a global FMD pandemic?

This is unlikely, unless the introduction of FMD into disease-free regions was malicious and targeted simultaneously to a number of different continents. Accidental incursion into a single country or geographic region is, however, a major and continuing risk. With regard to natural spread between continents, the main thing that quarantine authorities worry about is that FMD and other diseases like swine fever could be introduced in poorly heated meat products, particularly sausages.

As an island that has remained relatively free of the main veterinary diseases, Australia has very strict quarantine. That's the main reason, for example, that people deplaning after a 5–10 hour flight from Asia or 13+ hours from the Americas are likely to have their luggage X-rayed before they leave the customs hall. There are other motives, including the exclusion of illegal guns and other lethal weapons, but blocking the entry of diseases like FMD is the main economic justification. No matter where they come from, travelers will also be asked if they are carrying sporting gear (particularly for fishing) or have been on a farm recently. Answering in the affirmative may mean that your suitcase has to be unpacked so that walking boots and trout rods can be inspected and, if necessary, cleaned with disinfectant. The North American infectious hemopoietic necrosis virus of rainbow trout infects a number of salmonid species and, though it has so far been excluded from Australia, it has crossed to Asia and to Europe.

It's easy to imagine that a sporting tourist could transfer an infection to trout streams via contaminated boots or fishing gear, but how might a cow or a pig be exposed to a virus that's been imported in a sausage? The problem is that pigs, in particular, are often fed discarded organic material from restaurants. Proper heat sterilization will kill FMD, but the 2001 UK outbreak, for example, is thought to have resulted from inadequately heated, infected meat scraps that were fed to cattle on a single farm in Cumbria. The virus may then have spread rapidly around the country as a consequence of livestock movements (often illegal) between different properties and to abattoirs and sale yards.

Has an animal virus ever been introduced deliberately into "virgin soil"?

This has occurred at least twice in Australia. But both introductions were not malevolent, at least so far as people were concerned, though the consequences for rabbits were very bad indeed. It's worth talking about this because what happened ranks high among the best-studied examples of a virus pandemic. The objective was pest control, to deal with a massive and persistent rabbit plague. This should have been an epidemic rather than a pandemic, but as described below, the infection was introduced into a further WHO region as a consequence of human intervention.

Rabbits are not native to Australia and were first brought to the country at the time of European settlement (the First Fleet) in 1788. They did not establish in the wild in any great numbers, however, and caused no problem. Then, in 1859, thinking that he might make his new world a little more like "home" in England if he could enjoy a bit of shooting, Thomas Austin released a mix of 12 wild rabbits and some domestic rabbits on his property near Winchelsea in the southern state of Victoria. Others followed his example. With few predators, the rabbits multiplied and spread across the continent. By 1950, it was estimated that there were 600 million rabbits (and 8.3 million humans) in the country, compromising both the natural environment and the economy by competing for grass with sheep and cattle, damaging native habitats, and promoting soil erosion. Every attempt to reduce rabbit numbers, which included poisoning, shooting, and building "rabbit proof" fences, failed.

The idea of biological control came from an Australian medical scientist, Dame Jean MacNamara, who while traveling in the Northern Hemisphere had visited Richard E. Shope at his Rockefeller Institute laboratory in Princeton, New Jersey. Already a hero of infectious disease research for the first identification of an influenza virus (in pigs) in 1931, Dick Shope's scientific reputation became even bigger when he discovered in 1932 that a naturally occurring tumor of cottontail (*Sylvilagus*) rabbits is caused by a poxvirus (called Shope Fibroma). Not long after Jean MacNamara visited, Shope also published on the closely related myxomavirus that was later to cause the greatest rabbit wipeout in recorded history. First discovered as a cause of non-lethal skin tumors in cottontails from Uruguay, myxomatosis virus is extremely lethal for European (*Oryctolagus cuniculus*) rabbits.

Lobbying by Jean MacNamara led to experiments with myxomavirus in England and on Wardang Island in the

Spencer Gulf of South Australia. After establishing that there were no obvious risks for domestic animals and wildlife species, limited field trials were done in the dryer northern part of South Australia. But the virus failed to establish and died out in the wild. Still, the feisty Jean MacNamara was unconvinced and, after a hiatus when everyone was otherwise preoccupied during World War II, her aggressive advocacy saw to it that the idea of using myxomavirus to control the Australian rabbit plague was given a second chance. Spread by both direct contact and by fleas and mosquitoes that had fed on an infected rabbit, the more extensive release of myxomatosis in 1950 led to a massive, continuing, outbreak that killed more than 98% of infected wild rabbits.

This was an enormous triumph for what has become known as "biological control." At a time when the average yearly wage of a factory worker was less than £300, the value of the wool crop increased by some £30 million in the year following the "myxo" introduction. Jean MacNamara was given a reward of £800. She had already been made a Dame of the British Empire for her earlier work on poliomyelitis including (with Sir Macfarlane Burnet) the discovery that there is more than one strain.

In those early days, the evolution of the virus in nature was studied intensively by Canberra virologist Frank Fenner, who later served as chair of the WHO Committee that oversaw the global eradication of another, distantly related poxvirus infection of humans, smallpox. Over the years, more resistant rabbit strains emerged in Australia but, with a current mortality from myxomatosis at around 50%, the massive rabbit counts of the first half of the twentieth century have not been restored. That continued limitation of population size also reflects the 1995 introduction of rabbit hemorrhagic disease (RHD). Caused by a calicivirus that was first discovered in China and was in the process of being safety-tested on Wardang Island, the RHD virus escaped into the wild. Millions of rabbits were killed within a matter of months. As with myxomatosis, this calicivirus infection persists in Australian rabbit populations, but the level of resistance (and the wild rabbit count) is, again, rapidly increasing.

The preceding tells the "legal and planned" half of the rabbit biological control story, but there is another tale that reflects what happens when individuals take matters into their own hands. Wanting to control the wild rabbits on his property, retired French bacteriologist and academician Paul Armand-Delille got hold of some myxomavirus and injected two rabbits, which he then released at Chateau Maillebois in the Loire Valley. Armand evidently believed that the virus would be confined within the environs of his enclosed estate but, within weeks, a dead rabbit was found 50 km away, and the disease spread rapidly. By 1953, for example, domestic rabbits in Wales were dying in large numbers. Rabbits are valued in Europe, so this was a problem for both pet owners and for commercial breeders. Fortunately, Shope fibroma virus both causes a mild, recoverable disease in European rabbits and protects against later exposure to myxomavirus. Licensed for use as a vaccine in the Northern Hemisphere, concerns that it may establish in the wild have led to Shope fibroma virus being banned in Australia.

Armand-Delille may have made a mistake, but that certainly doesn't describe what happened later with the rabbit calicivirus in New Zealand. Following the accidental release in Australia, the New Zealand public health authorities conducted an extensive process of public consultation and came to the conclusion that they would not allow the release of the RHD calicivirus. Farmers are then thought to have taken matters into their own hands and, from 1998, the disease has been established in New Zealand wild rabbit populations. Of course, once RHD was in the country, no effort was made to control the spread of the infection and, in fact, the process of deliberate dissemination is thought to have continued. Obviously, the reaction would be very different if this had been one of the hemorrhagic fever viruses that infect humans.

Both the myxomatosis and the RHD rabbit introductions occurred in the context of a modern understanding of virus diseases. In a sense, though, they can also be thought to illustrate what happened in earlier (pre-1850) times, when new viruses came into fully susceptible human populations who had no understanding of the germ theory of infection and no access to therapeutic or preventive measures. The fate of these "closely watched rabbits" in Australia recalls the catastrophic consequences of introducing Old World infections (like measles and smallpox) into the New World of the Americas and the Pacific Islands, including the Australian and New Zealand indigenous communities. Fortunately, we now live in a global climate where, so far as that is possible, public science functions to protect humanity. At least since the nineteenth century, when there was some deliberate spread of smallpox to kill off native peoples, so far as we are aware there has been no malevolent dissemination of any human virus.

Other than as a consequence of bioterrorism, is a veterinary pandemic likely?

Yes, though it has not "gone global," this describes what has happened with hi-path avian influenza over the past decade or so. If you substitute birds for people and follow the WHO rule that a Level 6 pandemic must be declared when a novel virus variant causes widespread disease in more than one WHO region, then the spread of the avian H5N1 influenza A virus from East Asia to West Asia, the Middle East, North Africa, and Europe certainly qualifies for the domestic chickens and ducks of this world. Estimates of the numbers of birds that were either killed by this infection or culled range from about 200 million (with a cost of $10 billion) to 1 billion, and it isn't over yet. If the virus had "jumped" across species to cause a severe, global, human pandemic, a World Bank estimate puts the cost at about $300 trillion.

Zealous veterinary authorities are constantly on the watch for "exotic" avian flu strains, with regulators in Victoria, Australia, recently killing some 24,000 ducks following the detection (during routine testing) of a hitherto exotic, lo-path H5N1 influenza virus. This posed no immediate threat to avian or human health, but the concern was that it could mutate to greater virulence.

Another way to trigger an animal pandemic/panzootic would be to bring representatives of a species from all over the planet, hold them together for a time, and then return them to their countries of origin. That describes the situation for equestrian events at an Olympic Games, though the expectation would be that the horses are both vaccinated against known pathogens (especially influenza) and very closely monitored for any signs of disease, particularly respiratory.

Top racehorses travel regularly by air, though they are subject to quarantine. The 2007–2008 H3N8 equine influenza outbreak in Australia was likely triggered by imported Japanese racehorses. Somehow, the virus jumped from the quarantine station to horses pastured nearby and was then widely disseminated from a local race meeting. This virus also spread to a few farm dogs and, though H3N8 is endemic in dogs in the United States, the re-isolated strain was definitely of horse and not canine origin. Only about 8% of the Australian horse population was directly involved, so the decision was made to eradicate the infection. In all, the total economic cost to the horse industry was estimated at around $380 million, with about $340 million of that being compensated by the Australian federal government, which is responsible for animal quarantine.

In general, governments everywhere have been relaxing animal quarantine measures and are spending much less on resourcing veterinary diagnostic and research facilities. This may be a major mistake. Also, apart from the economic costs associated with disease incursions into domestic livestock and other high-visibility animals, there is the issue of pathogens that infect other less obvious, and often unloved, species like amphibians. The fad for "exotic pets" means that many animals that would normally have been left in their home territory, or held in zoos, are now being moved around the world to live in private houses and apartments.

Maybe the stories of alligators in New York sewers are apocryphal, but released Burmese pythons are certainly disrupting the ecology of Florida's Everglades. Such animal incursions that compromise the ecological niches and food sources of native species can have enormous, though often unmeasured, secondary impacts affecting, for example, the pollination of plants and insect control, both of which have economic consequences. We should be very concerned about the continuing spread of the *Batrachochytrium dendrobatidis* fungus, for example, which has wiped out many species of frogs. This horrible disease is thought to have originated in Africa, but is now global in distribution.

The recent, economically disastrous outbreak of a herpesvirus-like infection in Australian abalone could easily have been transmitted to other regions of the planet by the unregulated distribution of seafood. In 2011 alone, this disease is thought to have caused in excess of $5 million in revenue loss for abalone producers in South West Victoria, Australia. We take considerable care when it comes to monitoring the international movement of sausages, cattle, pigs, dogs, and horses but, with the increasing use of aquaculture, what happens with fish, mollusks (abalone, oysters), and crustacea (prawns/shrimp) must also be taken into account. All complex life-forms have their own spectrum of pathogens, and some, like the influenza A viruses of vertebrates, may cross between widely separated (in evolutionary terms) species.

We need to think beyond our species and the various large or cuddly mammals that are "poster species" for the conservation organizations. Rapid air travel, together with behavior patterns and economic strategies that take no account of broader consequences, are major risk factors when we consider the overall health of the global biota. That's true if we're thinking of plants or animals, ranging from mollusks and fish to mammals. We are currently experiencing the sixth major extinction of life-forms that has occurred during the long history of our planet. This is justifiably described as the first anthropogenic extinction. In our carelessness and obsession with short-term economic goals, we are the primary cause.

Are animal and human pandemics dealt with very differently?

Yes, they undoubtedly are. Restricting the movements of cows and abalone (if we decide to do that) is comparatively easy, but the situation has to be very dangerous indeed before we could even contemplate such actions with people. The cost of shutting down international air travel is so massive that we don't even do that if, say, a country is currently experiencing a severe, seasonal influenza outbreak. At the height of the SARS epidemic when the identity of the virus was still a mystery, travel from East Asia to the United States, Europe, Australia, and so forth was not blocked. Part of the reason is that by the time we realize there's a problem and move to "shut the stable door," the horse in question has likely bolted. Such was the case for the 2009 H1N1 SW flu.

That doesn't mean that we do nothing. Cabin crew are trained to be aware of passengers who are unwell, and arriving air travelers can be "channeled" past quarantine authorities who check for obvious signs of illness. As mentioned, at the time of SARS, devices that take the temperatures of incoming passengers were placed prominently in many airports. That was continued through the 2009 "swine" flu pandemic, but the experience so far is that the efficacy of thermal scanning is marginal, especially if the number of cases is low. Thermal scanners no doubt have an important psychological effect, though knowledge of their presence may also backfire if people take over-the-counter drugs that depress body temperatures and help to disguise symptoms while traveling, especially if they're not feeling too great and are trying to get home from some distant location. When it comes to an infection like influenza, we differ (both genetically and in other ways) in our level of susceptibility at any given time. Even those with a mild case of flu can bring back a virus that will cause severe disease in others.

Can returning tourists be infected with something that transmits to animals?

Yes, as we discussed, it is possible that the mosquito-transmitted West Nile flavivirus that can be lethal for humans, horses, and birds (especially crows and magpies) was introduced to New York City in the blood of a subclinically infected human traveler. Also, some of the larger parasites, like tapeworms, have complex life cycles that involve humans and other animals. These are not, however, likely to cause disease outbreaks, let alone pandemics. Similarly, while the H3N8 influenza A virus undoubtedly jumped from U.S. horses to establish as an endemic infection in American greyhounds and then other dog breeds, this influenza strain has not been found to infect humans. On the other hand, we do know that influenza viruses circulating in pigs can be essentially identical to those found in people. There may be a chicken-and-egg argument here as to who got what first, but the spread of a variant H3N2 virus from pigs to in-contact people at U.S. agricultural fairs during 2012 provides, as discussed in more detail in Chapter 4, a good example of how these dynamics can play out.

Can imported animals infect humans?

That could happen but, at least for mammalian species, transporting animals between continents generally involves thorough health checks and a period of quarantine where appropriate. Australia, for example, is free of rabies, while this disease is endemic in U.S. wildlife (raccoons, foxes). Pet dogs and cats that make the long flight south across the Pacific must have a valid rabies vaccination certificate and are quarantined for 30 days after arrival. Bringing your dog or cat to the Antipodes will cost you in the range of $1,000 to $1,500.

Of course, there are also concerns about the *illegal* importation of animals. One scenario to explain the 1999 West Nile virus incursion into the United States is that, after being smuggled into the country, an infected bird was bitten by a New York mosquito. Countries like Indonesia and Australia, for example, ban the export of native parrots. The result is an illegal trade in these species. Indonesian birds are generally sold from Singapore, which is readily reached by boat or land transit via Malaysia. But, for an isolated island nation like Australia, taking small birds (like budgerigars) out of the country often means that they have to be anesthetized in some way and then hidden under clothing. That practice has led to the colloquialism of "budgie smuggler" to describe a particularly brief form of male swim-gear. Parrots can carry the respiratory infection psittacosis, which caused a big scare and killed a few Americans around the time of the 1929–1930 stock market crash, but this bug is readily killed by antibiotics and would never cause a pandemic.

When it comes to amphibians and reptiles, these species can figure in the life cycle of a few insect-borne viruses that occasionally infect humans. Otherwise, though, apart from eating a filter feeder (oyster, clam) that has concentrated some human pathogen (hepatitis A virus) from sewage-contaminated seawater, viruses that infect cold-blooded species do not normally transmit to mammals. Infection with fungi and bacteria (especially *Salmonella* species) can be an issue if bitten by an "exotic" pet like a large lizard but, again, these cause individual problems that can be treated with antibiotics, and there is little likelihood of human-to-human transmission.

Can humans be infected from imported animal or other products?

Yes, of course: that's why pregnant women are advised to avoid some of the most delightful imported soft cheeses that, if inadequately sterilized, can carry *Listeria monocytogenes*, a bacterium that is known to cause fever and possible miscarriages. Salmonellosis commonly results from eating poorly cooked eggs and poultry products sourced from badly maintained production facilities, but such occurrences are usually limited to within a particular country or region and don't generally lead to human-to-human transmission.

In Summary

Pandemics, epidemics, and even infectious disease outbreaks that involve humans can cause major economic damage. That's also very true for veterinary pathogens, though in the absence of some malevolent act, it's unlikely that a veterinary disease will move beyond the geographical bounds of one or other continental landmass. In general, relaxing the current quarantine barriers on imported, risky food products and live animals is a bad idea, and the situation regarding imported marine and exotic pet species would undoubtedly benefit from more attention. The libertarian fantasy of an unregulated world is particularly toxic when it comes to quarantine and the international movement of various animal species. This should continue to be an important, priority area for responsible governments.

11

BIOTERRORISM

Could sophisticated terrorists initiate a pandemic?

Yes, that is a legitimate concern. Anything to do with those who are capable of extreme violence justified by delusional self-righteousness is dangerous. But the problem with deliberately starting a pandemic is that, by definition, rapidly spreading pathogens like the influenza A viruses go everywhere. Even if those who set the infectious process in motion take steps to ensure their own survival, can they hope to extend that protection to the broader community whose interests they claim to represent? Despite this fact, since September 11, 2001, and the events that unfolded around the world over the subsequent decade, many have the sense that extremist zealots are capable of almost anything, even if the attack strategy leads ultimately to their own destruction.

I'm not so convinced of that, personally. Those senior figures who influence the young to sacrifice their lives in the pursuit of some "righteous" cause invariably take care to avoid putting themselves in harm's way. Their rationalization is presumably that there is little point to the action if the core of the organization is wiped out and there are no leaders left to pursue the intended goal.

But, as the recent murders of health care workers in Pakistan and Nigeria illustrate, it is the case that we live in a time where the health of fellow citizens, including children, can be seen as less important than making one or other political statement. Bioterrorism is certainly taken very seriously by governments around the world, especially in those nations, like the United States, the United Kingdom, and Russia, that have suffered one or other major terrorist episode. The CDC lists some 150 infectious agents that could potentially be used as terror weapons. However, even if a terrorist cell can access the virus or bacterium in question, and some are not particularly hard to come by, the group needs the laboratory facilities and the technical sophistication to generate these organisms in volume. Beyond that, they must have the capacity to distribute the infection to large numbers of people. Finally, while many of these diseases may be terrible, they are not all that readily transmitted.

The transmission problem can be overcome on the battlefield by delivering large doses locally with bombs, rockets, or even, if the wind is in the right direction, some form of aerosol generator. But the general view is that biological weapons are, like the poison gas that was used in much the same way by armies in World War I, ultimately unacceptable in every sense. Apart from any view based in morality or ethics, their unpredictability means that most infectious agents just aren't particularly effective as either strategic or tactical weapons. Their main utility would be to create panic and a sense of terror. In contrast, even the remote possibility that such weapons could be used can serve as an excuse for those who wish to perpetuate a sense of fear as a justification for repressive political actions.

Militarily, there is no enthusiasm for biological warfare. While the United States, the United Kingdom, and Russia all had active biological weapons programs through World War II and the earlier part of the Cold War that followed, any efforts to manufacture, store, and test the distribution of such materials were brought to a final end in 1975 when the international Convention on the Prohibition of the Development, Production and Stockpiling of Bacteriological (Biological) and Toxin Weapons and on their Destruction came into effect. This was signed by 163 countries and, since then, any research efforts funded by major states have been concerned with protecting rather than attacking human populations.

What about Saddam Hussein and his weapons of mass destruction?

The fact that Saddam Hussein and his henchmen used poison gas to murder 3,000–5,000 men, women, and children in the Kurdish town of Halabja established beyond doubt that he had no respect for international law and that his regime was capable of any atrocity. As a consequence, intelligence reports suggesting that Saddam was sponsoring the manufacture and stockpiling of biological weapons certainly gave cause for legitimate concern. But after much searching, while there were indications that the regime had traveled a little way down that path in earlier times, no evidence was found of an active biological weapons program. Still, in my view, that is where the main threat of a bioterror-initiated pandemic lies, in the activities of some rogue state.

Why is a rogue state more worrisome than a terrorist cell when it comes to biological weapons?

While a sophisticated, small terrorist group might indeed mount some form of localized attack, perhaps along the lines of what happened in the United States with anthrax subsequent to 9/11, it's much harder to see how they could launch a selective pandemic that would spare those whose interests they are trying to advance. It is not impossible, but it is unlikely. One scary scenario raised by the former Russian bio-weapons scientist Ken Alibeck suggests that at least a few stocks of the "weaponized" infectious agents generated in the former Soviet Union were not destroyed and might fall into the hands of terrorists or some extortionist mafia. Again, would even the most irresponsible group launch a pandemic that has the potential to endanger their own families and communities? Of course, the concern here would be that the individuals involved might not be sufficiently aware of the risks and ignorant of the possible "flow-on" effect.

In general, though, to generate and manufacture a bioterror weapon that would cause substantial loss of life and fear worldwide while leaving a substantial segment of humanity (the chosen people) unaffected, it would be necessary to achieve a level of organization well beyond what might be expected for any small group. As we all realize, the reason that terrorist cells are able to survive is that they maintain effective isolation and avoid the use of electronic media. A structure of that type is no doubt ideal when it comes to delivering an unexpected blow, but it could not work in a situation where an infectious agent that spreads everywhere is the weapon of choice. Even in the worst case scenario that such a group gains access to, and uses, a tactical (battlefield) nuclear weapon in a major city, the physical effects of the explosion and subsequent fallout would be local rather than global, though the terror message would be felt by everyone on the planet.

That's why I think that any intent to deploy a pandemic terror weapon would necessarily have to originate from a rogue nation state. If, for instance, the plan was to use smallpox virus, it would first be essential to vaccinate the country's own population, together with identical ethnic groups, co-religionists, or whoever that happen to be located elsewhere. Smallpox vaccine (vaccinia) is not currently given to other than a few personnel in research laboratories, and the vaccination process (scarification into the arm) is not used to protect against any other pathogen. Even the most rudimentary and ineffectual intelligence apparatus could not fail to detect the widespread use of smallpox vaccine, and it is certain that this would alert those who "war-game" bioterror scenarios.

There is a caveat. Vaccinia, the live, attenuated virus (perhaps originating from cowpox) that was used to eradicate smallpox as a naturally occurring disease is both big and readily manipulated in the laboratory to serve as a "virus vector" for the delivery of genes from other pathogens, generally as part of some experimental immunization strategy. My own research group has, for example, used such engineered vaccinia strains to analyze immunity to components of several other viruses, including influenza. Both in subhuman primates and, to a much more limited extent in people, vaccinia strains that express HIV proteins have been trialed as potential (and to date relatively ineffective) immunogens. Such vaccinia vectors would, however, work very well to block smallpox infection. Their use for that purpose could be "hidden" by what was claimed to be a program to test a novel, genetically engineered vaccine virus that is ostensibly being trialed as a protection against something else.

Why would smallpox potentially be used in bioterrorism?

One of only two infectious agents that are considered to have been eliminated globally, the last natural case of smallpox was diagnosed in 1975, and the WHO declared that the world was free of this virus four years later. The net consequence, though, is that those born after the end of smallpox vaccination in the 1970s have no preexisting immunity. Also, by the 1960s, smallpox was increasingly limited to a few countries in the developing world, so Westerners were only vaccinated if they were traveling to places where the disease was still active. The majority of the human population is thus at risk, which is why smallpox virus (*Variola major*) is one of the agents that remains a concern to those responsible for public health and national defense.

Since 1979, almost all variola stocks have been destroyed, and those that remain (so far as is known) are stored under the highest security conditions. Still, there is a concern that smallpox virus may be held, perhaps unwittingly, in a deep freeze in some isolated, unknown laboratory. In addition, the sequence of smallpox virus is a matter of public record, and any sophisticated genetic engineer could effectively reconstruct this pathogen from some closely related virus. Both monkey pox and vaccinia, the smallpox vaccine virus, could supply appropriate "frameworks" for remaking this scourge of humanity.

Like vaccinia, variola is both easy to grow in the laboratory and hardy in the sense of being resistant to temperature/environmental effects. Aerosols of stocks grown to very high titer are known to have spread through air-handling systems, so it is only safe to work with this pathogen in the type of "contained" biosecurity facility found typically in certified, high-security laboratories. Given that such a resource is available, though, small, freeze-dried aliquots (batches) of white powder containing billions of infectious particles could easily be manufactured for surreptitious transport around the world. This technology is widely available. Freeze dryers are used commercially to produce long-life, lightweight food products, and in laboratories to preserve infectious organisms.

The disease is very infectious and would inevitably cause a new pandemic if released simultaneously at a number of geographic points throughout the globe. What protections are there? The first is that we have a long history of dealing effectively with this disease. The characteristic, dramatic skin lesions (pocks) are readily recognized clinically and as a consequence, all smallpox cases would be quickly isolated in any society that has a functioning public health service. Though a terrible disease, smallpox is not invariably lethal and, even at its worst and spreading under the poorest conditions of clinical care, nutrition, and hygiene, in excess of 60% of those infected survived. Also, while variola can spread via the respiratory route, that generally requires a substantial period of close contact, and people are not very infectious before the pocks become visible. Additionally, the vaccine is still available and given regularly to research personnel who work with engineered variants. Vaccinia has long been approved for human use, large amounts can be produced quickly, and stockpiles remain viable in the long term.

Even when smallpox still raged globally, any incursions into disease-free communities (like those in Australia) were quickly recognized, and the infection was contained by quarantine and vaccination. An organized, criminal reintroduction of smallpox could be terrible, not least because it would strike at the spirit of what has been one of humanity's greatest collective achievements, but it is reasonable to expect that an outbreak, even if it occurred in multiple sites, would be dealt with before too many lives were lost. The only concern might be that a novel "bioterror" version of variola had been engineered in some way to overcome the protection conferred by vaccination.

Some years back, warning bells sounded in the aware scientific community when genetic manipulation of the mouse equivalent, ectromelia virus, inadvertently produced a variant that was not blocked by prior immunization. Again, making such a virus requires a high degree of technical sophistication that would, for example, only be found in an established state or well-resourced private laboratory. Furthermore, unless this was a mass suicide strategy, the group responsible would also have to develop a novel, protective vaccine. Should there be any suspicion that such a product was being distributed, espionage agents might need to obtain serum from vaccinees so that lab scientists could determine whether their antibody profiles were unusual. Of concern would be the presence of antibodies that bind to vaccinia virus without neutralizing infectivity. Hopefully, such scenarios belong to novelists and Hollywood scriptwriters rather than to the real world.

What do we know about anthrax?

Shortly after 9/11, powdered material containing highly resistant anthrax spores was distributed through the U.S. Postal Service in envelopes addressed to a number of prominent individuals, including two U.S. Democratic senators, Tom Daschle and Patrick Leahy, both well-known liberals. The enclosed, brief notes carried the statement, "Allah is Great," in a too-obvious attempt to implicate Islamic extremists. In all, a total of 22 people were clinically affected, including a number who worked for the postal service, and 5 died.

This event confirmed that anthrax (*Bacillus anthracis*) is an extremely effective bioterror weapon, though even if it were to be distributed simultaneously in a number of countries, it would be unlikely to cause a pandemic in the conventional sense of the term. The use of the postal service does show how easily anthrax spores can be disseminated. Even so, if this happens again, the widespread availability of electronic communication, banking services, and so forth, would mean that any global shutdown of the mails would be much less disruptive than might have been the case in 2001. One consequence, however, is that the simple receipt of a letter containing a white or brown powder leads automatically to the evacuation of an office, or even a building, and is an immediate matter for police/forensic investigation. Talcum powder, gypsum, or flour are perfect materials for perpetuating a disruptive hoax, but anyone who does that risks suffering some very severe penalties.

The anthrax used in the 2001 attack was quickly identified as the Ames strain that is, or was, held in research laboratories throughout the world. By 2005, the massive FBI investigation had focused much of its attention on a bacteriologist, Bruce Ivins, working at the U.S. Army's Medical Research Institute for Infectious Disease (USAMRID) high-security facility at Fort Detrick, Maryland. Though I don't recall ever meeting Ivins, I have known a number of USAMRID scientists over the years, and have never been in any doubt that their basic role is to prevent, rather than cause, infections. In particular, service personnel and civilian researchers working at both USAMRID and at AFRIMS (Armed Forces Research Institute of Medical Research) in Thailand have done a great job with tropical infections like dengue fever.

Bruce Ivins committed suicide in 2008, so the case was never tested through the courts. The U.S. legal system operates on the presumption of innocence. While the evidence has been described as damning and the case has been closed, doubts continue to be raised, along with speculation about possible cover-ups and conspiracies. Was Ivins, or some hidden individual who has so far escaped detection, the classical Hollywood mad scientist? The possibility that some seemingly functional but deeply disturbed individual may have access to dangerous materials, whether they be toxins, microbes, or a nuclear trigger, is a continuing cause of concern.

Can you envisage other novel bioterror pandemic scenarios?

Lots, but I would hate to put speculations out there that might influence the thinking of some malevolent individual or group. One important message is that all those working with dangerous infectious agents need to remain watchful, both locally and globally, and to contact representatives of the security agencies if they have any real concerns. There is a natural tendency to protect colleagues. But, as anyone who has run a research operation knows, the vagaries of the human condition and the prevalence of odd behavior in this community that attracts individuals who can be both extraordinarily intense and, in a few cases, socially isolated, means that it is sometimes essential to act, even if only to protect people against themselves.

Without going into any specifics, one speculative "Hollywood" scenario might be that some group of "green" scientifically aware zealots could decide to depopulate the planet in order to protect the global environment and limit the consequences of anthropogenic climate change. Achieving a sustainable world should be a real concern for all of us, but we need to do that by promoting the universal values of equity, cooperation, restraint, innovation, and mutual respect.

Whether we are on the political Right or Left of major issues, we should not simply dismiss extremist rhetoric. It is important to listen carefully to what is being said. Anyone who had managed to struggle through *Mein Kampf* prior to the

Nazi party achieving power in the German federal election of 1933 should have been in no doubt concerning the intentions of *Time Magazine's* 1938 "Man of the Year," Adolf Hitler. Yet we continue to elect people who embrace extremist positions to government. When it comes to national and global stability, the threat of an infectious disease pandemic may not necessarily be the biggest risk that we face.

Is a bioterrorist-initiated pandemic unlikely?

Localized bioterrorism acting at the level of spreading anthrax spores through the mail, dropping botulinus toxin into a reservoir, or disseminating some virulent infectious agent via a building air conditioning system does seem a realistic threat. But when it comes to deliberately triggering a human infectious disease pandemic, my personal sense is that such an event would both be too complex to initiate (such as with smallpox) or too unpredictable in extent (like influenza). There are many less demanding, more readily achievable and proven strategies for generating massive media coverage. Overall, unless the confrontation is extremely bitter and operating at short range, terrorist acts tend to be as much concerned with directing attention to some perceived injustice or "righteous" cause as they are with harming other people. If some group of zealots ever succeeded in triggering an influenza pandemic, then the disease, not their perceived grievance, becomes the story. Surely, as with any psychopath, our budding bioterrorist will have a psychological need to be permanently at the center of the narrative.

12

PROTECTING HUMANITY FROM AND DURING PANDEMICS

Is there anything that I can do personally to limit the possibility of a dangerous pandemic?

While pandemics are by their nature unpredictable, there are some things worth considering when it comes to the issue of personal safety and responsibility. The first point is to be a safe international traveler so that you don't bring some nasty infection home with you. Protect yourself and you protect others. Though taking the available vaccines won't prevent infection with some novel pathogen, it will contribute toward ensuring that you enjoy a successful vacation or business trip, and it should also put you in a "think bugs" mind-set.

If, for instance, you are off to Africa for a wildlife safari, make an appointment at a travel clinic (or with your primary care physician) two to three months ahead of time to check your vaccine status and, if needed, receive booster shots to ensure that your antibody levels are high. Anyone who is visiting a developing country should make sure that he or she has indeed received the standard immunizations of childhood. Adolescents and young adults are much more likely to suffer severe consequences if, for instance, they contract commonplace infections like measles or mumps that have, because of herd immunity, become so unusual in Western countries that a minority of parents reject the collective responsibility of vaccinating their kids. If you're younger and your parents are (or were) into alternative lifestyles, it may be wise to ask them very directly about your personal immunization history. It's also likely that, even if you were vaccinated early on, your level of immunity will have declined greatly and you will benefit from further challenge.

Both possibilities will be covered if you go to a comprehensive travel clinic, as the doctors and nurses there will insist that you receive these shots (or a booster) if you don't have a documented recent history. Any vaccination schedule should ideally be completed at least 3 to 4 weeks ahead of boarding your flight, the time needed for the full development of immunity. But this is one situation where "better late than never" applies. Should it have slipped your mind until the last minute, you should be vaccinated nevertheless. Even if you've never had that particular vaccine before, some level of protection could be there within 5 to 10 days, and a boosted, existing response will cut in more quickly. A travel clinic will also sell you a Gastro (gastroenteritis, not gastronomy) kit containing antibiotics to counter traveler's diarrhea (generally a result of low-grade *E. coli* infection), something to decrease intestinal/gastric motility (*Imodium*), and sachets of salts to restore an appropriate fluid balance.

For the elderly, be aware of the decline in immunity that happens with age. You may not respond to vaccines as well as those who are younger, and you will be at greater risk from any novel infection. Depending on your proposed itinerary, it may also be essential to take anti-malarial drugs, which generally have to be started well ahead of arrival. Malaria is not the only mosquito-borne threat in tropical countries, so carry a good supply of insect repellant. In general, think about when and where you travel. Avoiding the hot, wet season in the tropics may be a good idea, both from the aspect that too much rain can limit access to interesting sites and because more standing water means more mosquitoes. Wearing long trousers, long-sleeved shirts, and shoes and socks helps to protect against being bitten (both by insects and by snakes), while also minimizing skin damage due to higher UV levels. Then, before you make your plans and again prior to embarking, check the relevant websites at the CDC, the WHO, and your own Department of Foreign Affairs (Department of State in the United States) for travel alerts.

Especially if they're off to Asia, many of my medical infectious disease colleagues travel with one or other of the antiviral drugs (*Relenza* and *Tamiflu*) that work against all known influenza strains. These require a prescription, but they're worth having at home anyway in case there is a flu pandemic. If that happens, the word will be out that influenza is raging and stocks in the pharmacies and drugstores will disappear very quickly. But don't rely on self-diagnosis if you took your *Tamiflu* with you to some exotic place; see a doctor. What you may think is flu could be malaria.

For those who may be sexually active with a previously unknown partner, carry prophylactics (condoms) and behave as responsibly as possible. Excess alcohol intake increases the likelihood that we will do something stupid. Dirty needles must be avoided, but don't inject drugs under any circumstances. Blood-borne infections with persistently circulating viruses (HIV and hepatitis B and C) are major risks, while insect-transmitted pathogens (dengue, Chikungunya, Japanese B encephalitis) can also be in the human circulation for 5–10 days. Apart from that, being caught with illegal drugs can land you in terrible trouble, particularly in some Southeast Asian nations. No matter what passport you carry, you are subject to the laws of the country. Be aware that rabies may be endemic and that animal bites in general can be dangerous.

Can you really trust a tattooist to use sterile needles? Even if the needles are clean, what about the inks? How can they be sterilized to ensure that they are not, as has been known to occur, contaminated with *Mycobacterium chelonae*, the cause of a nasty skin infection? And that was in the United States, not in some exotic location where there may be much nastier bugs around.

What if I become ill while traveling?

Seek help the same day: that is, immediately! The local medical professionals will be very aware of the infections that are circulating in their area. Your hotel operator or tour organizer should be able to arrange this. Should you become sick on the flight back, let the cabin staff know and they will make sure that medical help is available on landing and that the appropriate authorities are informed. If someone else is affected and all passengers have to be quarantined, then accept that with good grace and go along with the decision.

What if I develop symptoms after I return home?

Once you are home, depending on how the local health system operates, you will be able to consult your own primary care doctor or internist. Infections, particularly bacterial infections, can kill very quickly. The person you need to see at the earliest possible opportunity will be a graduate of a recognized, science-based, Western-style medical school. While you may have the sense that visiting an amiable and supportive homeopath, chiropractor, or traditional/natural medicine practitioner is helpful when it comes, for example, to the relief of some chronic malady or persistent pain, such people are not trained to use the power of science to deal with acute infections.

Consider: though we have derived some very good drugs (digitalis, quinine) from natural plant products, such traditional medicines were presumably available all through those centuries when the plague ravaged Europe. With an acute infection, the primary requirement is likely to be rapid treatment with prescription drugs, sophisticated laboratory diagnosis, and, perhaps, admission to an infectious disease ward.

There you will have access to the best available technology and will be cared for by doctors and nurses with years of relevant education and experience. Apart from working very hard through 5 to 7 years of university medical school, infectious disease physicians will have had a further 5 to 6 years of specialist training. Then there are a number of short (1–3 month), intensive courses available to registered nurses and doctors who are involved in the practice of tropical medicine. As with any profession, the more cases practitioners see, the more likely they are to come to the correct conclusions.

The most likely cause of high fever and debility if you've been in an endemic area is malaria, possibly a drug-resistant variant that is not touched by whatever product you were taking. Give your doctor a full history and, if necessary, raise the question of malaria, as most physicians in the Western countries rarely, if ever, see this disease. Malaria can kill you, fast. On the other hand, you could have been infected by one of the insect-borne viruses, perhaps without realizing that you've been bitten. That's why it is important to use repellent and, where possible, to sleep in screened rooms or under a bed net. If you do become febrile or suddenly feel very dull and out of sorts, ensure that both your doctor and those close to you are looking out for any signs of hemorrhagic and/or neurological disease. A severe headache, blurred or partially obstructed vision, a stiff neck or any degree of numbness/paralysis could be an early sign of viral or bacterial meningoencephalitis. Not all brain infections are insect-borne, with poliomyelitis and other enteroviruses being other possible causes.

If you come down with severe respiratory symptoms after you were traveling in an area where some exotic (to your home country) infection is known to be circulating, it is advisable, for obvious reasons, to avoid going to a doctor's waiting room or to a hospital emergency department. Call your doctor or, failing that, the emergency services. They may be able to arrange a home visit by an informed professional who can, if necessary, organize for you to be admitted to some type of high-care, high-security facility. It may also be necessary for family and those in close contact to be quarantined, but those are judgments that have to be made by a qualified and experienced public health officer. In an ideal world, there would be a well-publicized telephone number that you could call immediately in such circumstances. But resources are always limited, and there may be no such mechanism in place. When you go the travel clinic for your shots, ask the doctor: whom should I call if there is an emergency following my return?

Apart from being a responsible traveler, what else might I do?

Even if we never travel outside our own country, there are things that we can do to limit the likelihood of, or the damage caused by, a possible pandemic. But it's not easy: complacency in the absence of any obvious threat is pretty much the social norm. The need is to overcome that natural tendency and be prepared, at a number of levels. When it comes to potential pandemics, the primary protection of society rests in the continuation of a strong tradition of researching, diagnosing, and dealing with both established and novel infectious diseases.

Education is, as always, enormously important. Everyone should have a clear understanding of how viruses and other pathogens are transmitted. We also need to engage with the nature of infection and immunity, including the way that vaccines work and how we are all protected by maintaining a good level of herd immunity. It is essential, for example, that every child (and parent) should be aware of the basics of personal hygiene, particularly cough etiquette and hand sanitation.

What is equally important is to maintain high standards and adequate staffing in agencies responsible for international quarantine (both human and veterinary), and to ensure that the spectrum of public health activities that operate at every level of government continues to receive appropriate levels of support. In the United States, the primary federal arm is the Commissioned Corps of the U.S. Public Health Service

(USPHS) and the central laboratories at the CDC, Atlanta. This is an incredible national resource that operates also at the global level, monitoring, for example, outbreaks of Ebola in Africa and serving as a WHO Reference Center for influenza. Pandemics are, by definition, international, and there is no room for the narrow parochialism that sometimes dominates national politics.

With regard to this issue of "forward defense" beyond a country's natural borders, it is the case that the total cost of eradicating smallpox from the planet was recovered within about two years. Dealing with polio and measles in the same way would also lead to a major payoff. Supported by donations from governments, major corporations, and private philanthropy, the GAVI initiative, for example, is committed to saving people's lives and protecting children's health in the poor countries. As stated in UN Millennium Development Goal 4, the commonly available vaccines provide the cheapest and most effective mechanism for achieving that end.

At least in democracies, every adult citizen has the right to vote. All of us need to think carefully about both our own role and the basic responsibilities of government. When it comes to the next election, question candidates directly about the issues that concern you and vote accordingly. Put public health and pandemic preparedness on that list.

Public health is not primarily a private sector function, though medical scientists, diagnostic technicians, and infectious disease doctors do use a lot of products (gloves, masks, culture plates, high-tech equipment, lab reagents, and so forth) sourced from industry. If we are involved with a political party, there is the opportunity to make the point that this is one area of taxpayer-supported activity that has to be preserved, and even enhanced. The United States, for example, spends massive amounts on secret communications surveillance intended to frustrate any possibility of a terrorist attack. It is doubtful, however, if any group of terrorists could cause something as globally or even nationally lethal as the 1918–1919 influenza pandemic. Of course, if a malevolent group did choose to dis-seminate some highly infectious biological weapon, much of our front-line defense would rest with the public health services and the military.

Are there useful steps that I can take at the level of my local community?

Yes, particularly in the United States, where local democratic institutions are strong. Various public health activities devolve down to the state, the county, the municipality, school boards, and the like. If you have direct involvement at any of these local authority levels, raise the question of whether public health issues are receiving due attention. These responsibilities might, for example, range from spraying for mosquito control to rat catching, to ensuring access to the vaccines of childhood, to maintaining a regional diagnostic laboratory. The cases for such activities must sometimes be defended, even though the fundamental importance of these functions should be very obvious to most reasonable people.

When serving on a local council, school board, or workplace safety committee, find out whether there is a well thought-out pandemic preparedness plan. If not, make the effort to put that in place. These were developed, for example, during the H5N1 bird flu scare in the first decade of this century. We might also probe whether the strategies outlined in an established plan are still appropriate for current realities. Do the various responsible individuals understand their functions and have access to the necessary resources? Are they even aware that they have such roles? What are the lines of communication, both upward to state and federal authorities and outward to the broader community?

What should people monitor if a catastrophe strikes? Do they know their emergency radio band, or is it the intent to use cell phones, "Apps" on i-phones, and the like? How will school-teachers, police officers, EMT personnel, doctors, hospitals, and those involved in the distribution of food and medicines be resourced and deployed? What steps might be necessary to ensure the security and safety of the water supply? Are emergency drills ever practiced? Once the acute threat goes away, such plans are often forgotten and left to gather dust on a shelf. The price of freedom is eternal vigilance, and the same is true when it comes to protecting against the essential randomness of any infectious disease incursion.

How do I protect my family if a pandemic hits?

Know where the emergency band is on your radio. Ahead of time, institute the type of disaster preparedness that is advised for all natural catastrophes, like earthquakes, floods, or being snowed in. There are a number of official websites that can advise you on this, both in the general sense and from the aspect of the local availability and the suitability of various products. These are easy to find, and much of what they suggest is commonsense. The difference between the pandemic and earthquake scenarios is, though, that the phase of acute danger may persist for months rather than hours or days. At best, any individual action is only likely to get you through to the stage where the responsible authorities organize safe protocols for food supply and so forth.

An obvious step is to set aside a stock of long-life foods, clean drinking water, flashlights and batteries, warm clothing, and so forth. Every household should have a digital clinical thermometer. There is also a spectrum of medical supplies that may rapidly become unavailable. Liquid disinfectant, hand sanitizer, and disinfectant wipes are essential for any infection control kit, but it's important to know the constituents and to recognize that (unless combined with benzalkonium chloride) alcohol-based products may be relatively ineffectual against some viruses (noroviruses, though not influenza). Paper towels and disposable tissues are also obvious components. Having a box or two of latex gloves like those used by medical professionals is worthwhile, but check stored items regularly, as they can deteriorate. Plastic bags are useful for sealing off contaminated waste.

There isn't a whole lot you can do concerning specific drugs. Most proprietary cold and flu medicines will, at best, only provide symptomatic relief, though it is important to have some alternative to aspirin available for young children. Drug stores also carry oral rehydration kits, which should last indefinitely. These contain salts that, when mixed at the specified concentrations in water and taken by mouth, correct the physiological imbalance resulting from massive fluid loss in, for example, severe diarrhea.

If an infection is raging, the first, obvious point is to be guided by the public health services. Consult government websites and listen to the advice being given by the responsible authorities on TV and radio. Avoid dubious information sources and "opinion makers" who may be in thrall to commercial interests, extremist political agendas, or just plain barking mad. Your favorite radio "shock jock" may be a skilled entertainer who speaks to your personal preferences, but the need here is to listen to serious people who have a level of responsibility and know what they're talking about. Follow advice on appropriate actions. Depending on the situation and the timing, the primary courses of action may be, on the one hand, for people to maintain effective social isolation or, on the other, to report to designated clinics and/or hospitals for diagnosis or treatment.

Regrettably, especially if we are experiencing a pandemic caused by some completely novel infectious agent, effective drugs and vaccines are not likely to be available. When it comes to prophylaxis (prevention), any stockpiled drugs, like the influenza antivirals that were purchased by governments at the time of the H5N1 bird flu scare, will be given first to those in the front line: customs and quarantine officers, police, medical personnel, food suppliers, and so forth. The same will be true for the initial doses of a new vaccine. My personal view is that the anti-vaccine sentiment that is so strong in some communities will go out the window in the face of a rapidly spreading, severe pandemic, especially if children are affected. People will be angry because vaccines are rationed and they do not have access to them.

Even so, should the problem be familiar, as would be the case with an extremely virulent, pandemic influenza A virus that has just jumped from pigs (or birds) into us, technologies that are just now becoming available will likely mean that a lot of vaccine can be produced and deployed very quickly. That will not be the case for something totally new, unless the relevant authorities, like the U.S. FDA, are prepared to bypass the full spectrum of normal safety testing through Phase 1 (safety) to Phase 3 (broad efficacy) trials. Risk-benefit analysis in the face of a rapidly spreading horror virus would likely suggest that if, for example, the vaccine is composed of a single viral protein made by standard recombinant DNA protocols, it would be out in the community after very limited evaluation.

In general, those who object to vaccines, who attack the integrity of the companies that make them, and who seek to degrade the capacity of the regulatory authorities that oversee their safety and use (like the FDA) might reflect a little and ask the question: "If we damage our vaccine development and production capacity, where will we be if humanity is hit with a severe pandemic caused by a novel pathogen?" Such resources take years to put in place and cannot be casually resurrected from nothing. Vaccines are part of our national defense, and they should be regarded as such by both the public and the politicians.

Encouraging cough etiquette is a good thing to do ahead of time. Spitting in the street is unacceptable, though it may be a social norm is some cultures. Rigorous hand washing with soap and water is of proven value. Evidence of efficacy is much less established for the type of face masks that are likely to be generally available to the broader public. Individual N95 respirators, like those worn by workmen to prevent dust inhalation, may be useful, but they aren't perfect. They reduce the likelihood of contracting, or transmitting, infection, but the only really safe mask is a respirator with an independent, filtered air supply. Relying on devices that tend to be hot, uncomfortable, and cumbersome is also fraught with the possibility of compromise due to human error. In many Asian countries, a face mask can be a sign that someone currently has a respiratory infection and is trying both to warn others and to minimize the possibility that the disease is passed on.

An obvious protective measure is to stay away from crowded places and public transport. Should you feel ill, don't go to school or to your workplace. Most people, in the advanced countries at least, are better off with regard to avoiding close contact than was the case for our ancestors during the 1918–1919 influenza pandemic. Inhabiting larger living spaces and with access to our own cars, it is much easier for us to maintain an effective social distance. The availability of e-mail and the Internet means that many can now work from home and do not need to go to school or to the office.

Local authorities may move rapidly to shut down schools and day care centers. This obvious strategy will have little useful effect if, for example, parents head off to work and the kids are brought together so that they can be looked after in one household. If you have an isolated country house and there are no travel bans, this might be a good time to take an extended vacation. Make sure you have a good Internet connection. In the end analysis, the basic essential is for everyone to understand how the infection in question is spreading and to be aware of any simple, basic steps that can be taken to minimize risk. Knowing the facts and understanding the intent behind various rules and recommendations is the best protection for reasonable, responsible people.

Does the idea of being "too clean" apply to pandemics?

No, not really: what we're talking about in the "too clean" context is the idea that normal environmental infections "train" a child's developing immune system. While it is important to cultivate sound hygiene practices within the family and to ensure that everyone has a good practical understanding of the nature of both infection and disease spread, that should not be paralyzing. Little kids, for example, need to get "down in the dirt."

The basic idea behind the "too clean" hypothesis is that early exposure to some of the infections and infestations suffered by humans through evolutionary time help to "skew" immunity down pathways that minimize the development of, for example, asthma following exposure to pollens or house dust mites. Children who live in "traditional" cultures are much less likely to be asthmatic than those who grow up in "first world" environments. One possibility would be to give a dose of roundworm eggs to every child who lives in a Manhattan apartment. Woody Allen could no doubt make something of that, and maybe the kids are the ones who really know the score. Some of us may remember the rhyme:

Nobody loves me, everybody hates me
Think I'll go and eat worms
Long ones, short ones, fat ones, thin ones
See how they wriggle and squirm. . . .

The same possibility is being discussed in regard to treating some forms of autoimmunity, particularly Crohn's disease. In the long term, a better idea may be to continue working out the underlying science so that we can deliver some product that's a bit less awful than worm bits.

Even so, while the young may need to encounter "environmental" bugs and bacteria, there is no excuse for their not receiving the vaccines that counter the potential killers of childhood. Whooping cough, diphtheria, measles, tetanus, and so on can all be very bad diseases, with long-term complications. The best advice is to be sensible, be thoughtful, respect evidence ahead of opinion and fantasy, and be aware. When it comes to infectious diseases, it's not about what we "feel." What matters is what we think and what we do.

Where do I look for help if I become infected during the course of a major pandemic?

If it is early and there are as yet few cases in your town or country, the whole medical apparatus is likely to be focused on identifying and, if possible, treating you. But, if the disease is widely established, medical personnel are exhausted (or sick themselves), and the overall situation is dire, all that may be available is the advice provided on authoritative websites. Then you will need to go along with whatever strategy is being recommended by public health officials. You may be able to make personal contact with a professional via call-in/texting to a designated "hotline." And, as discussed earlier, stick with the advice of doctors and other practitioners trained in the science-based Western tradition. During the severe 2012–2013 winter flu outbreak, hospitals in locations as diverse as Philadelphia and Peru established temporary tented facilities—heated in Philadelphia—to deal solely with cases of respiratory infection.

In the event that the hospitals and other medical services are overwhelmed, stay quiet, avoid alcohol intake, keep hydrated, and take every possible step to avoid passing the infection on to family and to others close to you. Don't assume that because someone is young and fit he or she may not develop severe disease. Particularly in emerging pandemics, the worst forms of influenza can be seen in those who are in robust good health and, as a consequence, make very strong immune responses. The ultra-fit can be more susceptible to cytokine-mediated shock, a condition that has the potential to kill very rapidly.

If you do become ill and then recover, you are likely to be permanently immune and potentially of great help if the disease is still active. First make sure, though, that what you experienced was indeed caused by the infection that's circulating. Such judgments need to be made professionally. If an appropriate diagnostic test does show that you're in the clear, then you can help care for the sick with impunity. It will also be the case that your serum is likely to contain high titers of antibody that may be of value if given to others for protective or therapeutic purposes. Also, if you were infected very early in the course of the pandemic, scientists may want to take a few of your white blood cells to provide the genetic material for making human monoclonal antibodies. Such reagents can ultimately be produced in large quantities and used in the same way as immune serum.

The Bottom Line

Don't panic, act sensibly, and listen carefully to what the responsible authorities are saying. Otherwise, without knowing the actual problem, it is impossible to develop hard and fast rules on what to do in the face of a pandemic infection. Obviously, it's important to be very aware of the various warnings and recommendations put out by public health authorities. Here, our cell phones, iPads, and computers give us an enormous advantage over earlier generations, providing we stick with responsible information sources and don't get drawn into some of the dissembling and collective weirdness that any of us can find anytime via the web or the radio dial.

While the propagation of fear and a sense of outrage concerning the actions of others can be a prime characteristic of some media "personalities" and organizations, neither is useful. Through history, one of the least attractive aspects of humanity has been the tendency to look for scapegoats. In medieval times, Jews, isolated women, and any who happened to be different were quite erroneously blamed for spreading the plague. Nobody targeted the rats and the fleas. Today, even if some bioterrorist cell did succeed in initiating a pandemic, that doesn't mean that innocent people who follow the same, broad religious tradition, for example, are in any way to blame. Forget conspiracy theories and think about survival rather than assigning blame. If some human agency bears a measure of responsibility for what has happened, that will inevitably come out in retrospect. Leave judgment to the law of the country.

Bear in mind that two of the worst pandemics of the twentieth century, HIV and hepatitis C, developed slowly and, initially at least, received little attention. Though some may be personally offended by, for example, homosexuality and "sexual liberation," it is essential that such value judgments do not compromise our capacity to deal with an emerging infectious disease pandemic. If providing condoms, clean needles, supervised drug injection facilities, judgment-free medical care, and the short-term restriction of movement for those who are not competent will help to minimize disease spread, then it is good public health policy to do so. Think pragmatically in terms of causality rather than belief. If you have a public voice on such issues, speak out in favor of evidence-based approaches.

As with any "natural" disaster, preparedness at the level of having a store of basic food and other supplies on hand is likely to be a good idea. That doesn't mean going to the extremes of "survivalist" mode. Otherwise, a few simple precautions remain our best line of defense. If, as is very likely, the disease is spread via droplet/aerosol inhalation, it's important to maintain personal distance and to avoid crowded spaces like movie theaters and shopping malls. That's especially the case with children, where isolation can pose particular difficulties, but children are often the optimal "multipliers" of any infection. Thinking "bugs everywhere" and being vigilant minimizes the level of risk. Hand washing/sanitization is important, as is cough etiquette and avoiding habits like nose picking and eye rubbing. So far as possible, make a practice of not touching your hands to your face. Much of what can be done is, in fact, just a matter of common sense.

13

CONCLUSIONS

The following summarizes key points and provides short comments on a few issues that come up in any discussion of global infectious disease.

- Modern air travel links us all in a very immediate, physical way. Any pathogen that spreads readily from human to human (particularly by aerosols) can no longer be confined to a particular landmass. While that may have been the case before the great explorations led by sailors like Christopher Columbus and James Cook, even slow movement by sailing ships led to situations in which novel infections, like measles and smallpox, had disastrous consequences for previously isolated indigenous populations. Now, we live much closer together on this small planet than we might sometimes wish to think.
- HIV taught us that a pathogen that may not be particularly infectious and requires sexual or blood transmission may initially be very limited in distribution, but with changing realities (rapid air travel, relaxation of sexual taboos) might suddenly emerge as a major pandemic.
- Humanity has experienced "fast" (influenza), "slow" (HIV), "needle" (hepatitis C), "below the major alert radar" (norovirus), and "ocean-limited" (Chikungunya) pandemics.

- Mutants of viruses currently circulating throughout the human family can emerge locally to spread globally. This happens with seasonal influenza, though, by convention, such occurrences that involve variants of familiar flu strains are not described as pandemics. The nomenclature situation may be different for the noroviruses.

- While there are a few situations, like MDR TB, where a pandemic pathogen could potentially emerge from within the human population, this generally happens when a natural infection of some wildlife or domestic animal species crosses over to infect us.

- To date, all human pandemics have been caused by pathogens that infect one or other species of warm-blooded vertebrate. There may be an insect vector involved, but that will inevitably limit the geographic distribution of the disease.

- Pathogen crossovers from one species to another are inherently random and unpredictable, though some known reservoir populations (like swine in the case of the influenza A viruses) merit close monitoring.

- The level of risk is increased when rapid forest clearing, odd culinary practices, and adventurous lifestyles bring wildlife species and humans in close contact.

- Completely novel infections that switch species to initiate pandemics tend to be relatively innocuous, or at least not acutely lethal, in their maintaining hosts, representing an evolutionary equilibrium that allows prolonged virus excretion while the animal in question remains mobile and spreads the disease.

- A window to historical times when measles and smallpox caused "virgin soil" epidemics in human populations native to the Pacific region and the Americas was opened for us when myxomavirus was deliberately released in 1950 to control Australian rabbits in the wild. With emerging resistance and recovering rabbit numbers, that process was repeated 45 years later with a hemorrhagic calicivirus.

In both cases, the initial consequence was massive death rates in wild rabbit populations. However, the evolution of genetic resistance driven by natural selection ultimately led to gradually increasing rabbit numbers, though the "rabbit plagues" seen prior to 1950 have not recurred.

- No pandemic is likely to wipe out the human species. Even without the protection provided by modern science, we survived smallpox, TB, and the plagues of recorded history. Way back, when human numbers were very small, infections may have been responsible for some of the genetic "bottlenecks" inferred from evolutionary analysis, but there is no formal proof of this.

- As seen following the 1918–1919 influenza catastrophe, pandemic pathogens tend to evolve to lesser virulence with time. That process of natural selection is, however, blocked when (as with HIV/AIDS) we limit death rates by protecting those who are infected with drugs. At least in that context, Western society at least is in a compassionate, "post-evolution" phase.

- Once established in a population, viruses rarely change their mechanism of spread. An exception is the influenza A viruses in birds, where lo-path strains that are normally excreted via the GI tract can mutate to give hi-path viruses that infect the lung and brain.

- What influenza also tells us is that, while viruses that spread via the respiratory route are the most likely cause of some future pandemic, only the most draconian and immediate restrictions on human travel are likely to limit the spread of infection, and then only briefly.

- Such limitations are likely to be applied quickly if we are faced with a situation in which, for example, more than 30% of those infected develop severe or even fatal consequences. The more dangerous situation may be when mortality rates are in the 1–3% range, causing (ultimately) 70 million to 210 million deaths globally. Such an infection could "get away" before we realized what was happening.

- While we endured two murderous world wars and repeat episodes of deliberate genocide (Nigeria, Rwanda, Cambodia), as well as the 1918–1919, 1957, 1968, and 2009 influenza pandemics, the HIV/AIDS pandemic, the hepatitis B and C virus pandemics, and so forth, the size of the human family increased more than fourfold over the interval 1900–2012. Infectious diseases undoubtedly served to limit human numbers before the modern scientific era but, unless we have massive social disruption due to some other cause, my personal view is that this is unlikely to be the case in the future.
- Though it may be counterintuitive in some senses, the best way to stabilize human population size is to educate and empower women, solve problems like malaria and tuberculosis, promote global prosperity, and achieve the UN Millennium goal of providing the standard vaccines of childhood for all. Especially in traditional agricultural societies, people cannot be expected to limit family numbers if they do not know that their children will survive.
- Our capacity to deal with and live through pandemic situations is continually improving. We should not be fearful, but we should be aware, watchful and prepared.
- There are steps that we can take to protect ourselves, our families, and our communities, but these need to be thought through ahead of time. Fostering sound personal habits related to cough etiquette, hand/face contact, and hand sanitation is a good place to start.
- As with any form of defense, it takes political will and financial resources (both public and private) to maintain the integrity of national borders (quarantine), support the professionals who serve in the public health field services and laboratories, and fund the research that leads to greater diagnostic acuity, novel drugs, and improved vaccines.

- Infectious diseases are no respecters of wealth, power, or personal merit. Pandemic infectious disease is one situation where we cannot accept Margaret Thatcher's view that "there is no such thing as society." With a fast-spreading respiratory virus, for example, everyone is ultimately in the same boat.

FURTHER READING

Books

The following lists a few books that deal with relevant infectious disease topics and, in some cases, tell dramatic stories about both the people and the risks associated with such work.

Alibek, K., and Handelman, S. *Biohazard: The chilling true story of the largest covert biological weapons program in the world—told from inside by the man who ran it*. New York: Random House, 2000. An account of what was happening in Russia during the Cold War.

Barry, J. M. *The great influenza: The story of the greatest pandemic in history*. New York: Viking Press, 2004. The most recent, comprehensive account of the 1918–1919 Spanish flu pandemic, with special emphasis on the state of U.S. medicine and biomedical research at that time.

Bazin, H. *The eradication of smallpox: Edward Jenner and the first and only eradication of a human infectious disease*. London: Academic Press, 2000. Strong on the history of smallpox.

Crosby, A. W. America's *Forgotten pandemic: The influenza of 1918*. 2nd ed. Cambridge: Cambridge University Press, 2003. This excellent account was the first (in 1976) to bring the 1918–1919 pandemic back into the broader consciousness.

Doherty, P. C. *Their fate is our fate: What birds tell us about our health and our world*. New York: THE EXPERIMENT, 2013. Also published in

Australia and New Zealand as *Sentinel chickens: What birds tell us about our health and the world*. Melbourne: Melbourne University Publishing, 2012. Expands on the avian influenza and West Nile virus stories and further discusses the interface between humans and the natural world when it comes to infection, poisons, planetary warming and habitat degradation.

Eron, C., 1981. *The virus that ate cannibals*. New York, Macmillan. Easy to read "detective stories" about some of the great pioneers of infectious disease research.

Garrett, L. *The coming plague: Newly emerging diseases in a world out of balance*. New York: Penguin, 1994. A journalist's classic account of emerging infections.

Geison, G. L. *The private science of Louis Pasteur*. Princeton, NJ: Princeton University Press, 1995. A readable account of the great pioneer.

Henderson, D. A., and Preston, R. *Smallpox—the death of a disease: The inside story of eradicating a worldwide killer*. Amherst, NY: Prometheus Books, 2009. How smallpox was eradicated, by the man who ran the WHO program.

Kaufmann, S. *The new plagues: Pandemics and poverty in a globalized world*. London: Haus Publishing, 2009. Reflecting his interests as a leading international researcher, Kaufmann is very good on bacterial and protozoal diseases.

Knipe, D. M., and Howley, P. M., eds. *Field's virology*. 5th ed. Philadelphia: Wolters Kluwer Health Lippincott Williams & Wilkins, 2006. The standard, authoritative text on virology.

Kolata, G. *The story of the great influenza pandemic*. New York: Touchstone, 1999. A popular account by a leading *New York Times* science journalist.

Mims, C. *The war within us: Everyman's guide to infection and immunity*. London: Academic Press, 2000. A very readable discussion of infectious disease by a former professor of microbiology.

Mullis, K. *Dancing naked in the mind field*. New York: Pantheon, 1998. An entertaining read from a very unusual Nobel Prize winner.

Oldstone, M. B. A. *Viruses, plagues and history*. New York: Oxford University Press, 1998. A sympathetic account by a leading research virologist, who also discusses some of the key historical figures.

Offit, P. A. *Deadly choices: How the anti-vaccine movement threatens us all*. New York: Basic Books, 2011. A very important book for anyone who is confused about the safety and value of childhood vaccination.

Pepi, J. *The origin of AIDS*. Cambridge: Cambridge University Press, 2011. Reviews how this virus emerged to cause a global pandemic.

Piot, P. *No time to lose: A life in pursuit of deadly viruses*. New York: W. W. Norton, 2012. A personal account from the medical scientist who tracked down Ebola, then founded and directed UNAIDS.

Preston, R. *The demon in the freezer: The terrifying truth about the threat from bioterrorism*. London: Headline Book Publishing, 2002. Scary monsters and horror scenarios.

Quammen, D. *Spillover: Animal infections and the next human pandemic*. New York: W. W. Norton, 2012. A well-known author tells human and science stories of what happens when viruses like Hendra jump the species barrier and infect us.

Wolfe, N. *The viral storm: The dawn of a new pandemic age*. New York: Time Books, Henry Holt, 2011. A scientist discusses how and why viruses crossover from animal reservoirs into human populations, and also addresses advances in technology that facilitate diagnosis and, perhaps, the possibility of prediction.

More background reading

The list that follows is by no means comprehensive. In the biomedical area, the U.S. National Library of Medicine *PubMed* database is open to everyone (http://www.ncbi.nlm.nih.gov/pubmed/). All you need from the references listed below is the first author's surname and initials, followed by the publication date. For example, to find: Leroy, E. M., et al. Fruit bats as reservoirs of Ebola virus. *Nature* 438: 575–5876, 2005, enter: "Leroy EM 2005.". That should take you to everything published by that author in that year, though you will also pick up papers from others with the same name. Omit the "2005" and you will see a lifetime record, including more recent articles. Sometimes a particular journal article can be downloaded in full; sometimes you will be charged, but you may think that it's important to read more than a 150–250 word abstract.

With the Public Library of Science (*PLoS*) online journals, the publisher recovers the cost up front and the material is "open access" for all to see. Those PLoS formats that are likely to contain articles of interest in the present context are *PLoS One, PLoS Medicine, PLoS Pathogens,* and *PLoS Tropical Neglected Diseases*. Additionally, there is a spectrum of open access journals published by BioMed Central (http://www.biomedcentral.com/journals), including *BMC Infectious Disease, BMC Microbiology, BMC Public Health,* the *Virology Journal,* the *Malaria Journal, Population Health Metrics,* and so forth.

But if you want rapid access to more information about a given infection, a past pandemic event, a vaccine, or a drug, the easiest place to start is often with *Wikipedia*. My experience with *Wikipedia* for infectious disease topics that I do know well is that the material presented is usually both comprehensive and reliable. Additionally, especially with regard to pandemics and global infectious disease, a great deal of useful information can be accessed via the U.S. CDC website (www.cdc.gov/). If you're off on vacation, the first thing that comes up is Traveler's Health section (http://wwwnc.cdc.gov/travel), which leads to information on the disease problems that may be prevalent in the area that you're visiting and advises on appropriate vaccinations. And the WHO also provides an enormous amount of up to date information on what's happening globally (http://www.who.int/topics/infectious_diseases/en/). Hopefully, the present book will help you to navigate through some of that information.

AIDS

Cohen, J. Halting HIV/AIDS epidemics. *Science 334*: 1338–1340, 2011.

Cohen, J., and Shelton, D. HIV treatment as prevention: ARVs as HIV prevention, a tough road to wide impact. *Science 334*: 1628 and 1645–1646, 2011.

Fauci, A. S. AIDS: Let science inform policy. *Science 333*: 13, 2011.

Feidi, R. A., et al. Dimeric 2G12 as a potent protection against HIV-1. *PloS Pathogens 6*: e1001225, 2010.

Gilbert, P. B., et al. Statistical interpretation of the RV144 HIV vaccine efficacy trial in Thailand: A case study for statistical issues in efficacy trials. *J. Infect. Dis. 203*: 969–975, 2011.

Hütter, G., and Ganepola, S. Eradication of HIV by transplantation of CCR5- deficient hematopoietic stem cells. *The Scientific World J. 11*: 1068–1076, 2011.

Korber, B., et al. Timing the ancestor of the HIV-1 pandemic strains. *Science 288*: 1789–1796, 2000.

Sattenau, Q. J. A sweet cleft in HIV's armour. *Nature 480*: 324–325, 2011.

Shattock, R. J., Warren, M., McCormack, S., and Hankins, C. A. Turning the tide against HIV. *Science 333*: 42–43, 2011.

Wadman, M. Cutbacks threaten HIV gains. *Nature 480*: 159–160, 2011.

Zhang, J., et al. Retroviral restriction factors TRIM5 alpha: Therapeutic strategy to inhibit HIV-1 replication. *Curr. Med. Chem. 18*: 2649–2654, 2011.

Bats, insects, rodents and hemorrhagic pathogens

Breed, M. F. F., et al. Evidence of endemic Hendra virus infection in flying-foxes (Pteropus conspicillatus): Implications for disease risk management. *Plos One 6*: e28816, 2011.

Feldmann, H., and Geisbert, T. W. Ebola haemorrhagic fever. *The Lancet 377*: 849–862, 2011.

Gowen, B. B., and Holbrook, M. R. Animal models of highly pathogenic RNA viralinfections: Hemorrhagic fever viruses. *Antiviral Research 78*: 79–90, 2008.

Halpin, K., et al. Pteropid bats are confirmed as the reservoir hosts of henipaviruses: A comprehensive experimental study of virus transmission. *Am. J. Trop. Med. Hyg. 85*: 946–951, 2011.

Hanna, J. N., Carney I. K., Smith, G. A., et al. Australian bat lyssavirus infection: A second human case, with a long incubation period. *Med. J. Aust. 172*: 597–599.

Jamieson, D. J., et al. Lymphocytic choriomeningitis virus: An emerging obstetric pathogen. *Am. J. Obstet. Gynecol. 194*: 1532–1536, 2006.

Leroy, E. M., et al. Fruit bats as reservoirs of Ebola virus. *Nature 438*: 575–5876, 2005.

Pulmanausahakul, R. Chikungunya in Southeast Asia: Understanding the emergence and finding solutions. *Int. J. Infect. Dis. 15*: E671–E676, 2011.

Yu, X.-Y., et al. Fever with thrombocytopenia associated with a novel Bunyavirus in China. *New Engl. J. Med. 364*: 1523–1532, 2011.

Bioterrorism and laboratory safety

Dellaporta, T. Laboratory accidents and breeches in biosafety: They do occur! *Microbiology Australia 29*; 62–65, 2008. http://www.theasm.org.au/uploads/pdf/MA_May_08.pdf.

Doherty, P. C., and Thomas, P. G. Dangerous for ferrets: Lethal for humans? *BMC Biology 10*:10, 2012. http://www.biomedcentral.com/1741-7007/10/10.

Domaradaskij, I. V., and Orent, W. Achievements of the Soviet biological weapons programme and implications for the future: *Rev. Sci. Tech. 25*: 153–161, 2006.

Jackson, R. J., et al. Expression of mouse interleukin 4 by a recombinant ectromelia virus suppresses cytotoxic lymphocyte responses and overcomes genetic resistance to mousepox. *J. Virol. 75*: 1205–1210, 2001.

Merka, T. J., et al. Development of a highly efficacious vaccinia-based dual vaccine against smallpox and anthrax, two important bioterror entities. *Proc. Natl. Acad. Sci. USA. 107*: 18091–18096, 2010.

Nordmann, B. D. Issues in biosecurity and biosafety *Int. J. Antimicrob. Agents 36*: S1, S66–S69, 2010.

Rasko, D., et al. Bacillus anthracis comparative genome analysis in support of the Amerithrax investigation. *Proc. Natl. Acad. Sci. USA 108*: 5027–5032, 2011.

Sandstrom, G., et al. A Swedish/European view of bioterrorism. *Ann. NY Acad. Sci. 916*: 112–116, 2000.

Common cold research unit

A short film of what went on there can be found at: http://www.britishpathe.com/video/common-cold-research-unit-salisbury.

Drugs and drug resistance

Farnia, P., and Behesti, S. Totally drug resistant TB strains: Evidence of adaption at the cellular level. *Eur. Resp. J. 34*: 1203, 2009.

Sugaya, N., et al. Long-acting neuraminidase inhibitor lanamivir octanoate (CS-8958) versus Oseltamivir as treatment for children with influenza virus infection antimicrob. *Agents Chemother. 54*: 2575–2582, 2010.

Wright, A., and Zignol. M. Rapporteurs: Anti-tuberculosis drug resistance in the world. WHO Report Number 4, pp. 1–142, 2008. Available online at www.who.int/topics/tuberculosis/en/.

Zignol, M., et al. Modernizing surveillance of antituberculosis drug resistance: From special surveys to routine testing. *Clin. Infect. Dis. 52*: 901–906, 2011.

Economics and the human/animal equation

Barber, L. M., Schleier, J. J., III, and Peterson, R. K. D. Economic cost analysis of West Nile Virus outbreak, Sacramento County, California, USA, 2005. *Emerg. Infect. Dis. 16*: 480–486, 2010.

Curley, M., and Thomas, N. Human security and public health in Southeast Asia: The SARS outbreak. *Aust. J. International Affairs 58*: 17–32, 2004.

Hehme, N. Influenza vaccine supply: Building long-term sustainability. *Vaccine 26S*: D23–D26, 2008.

Molinari, N. A., et al. The annual impact of seasonal influenza in the US: Measuring disease burden and costs. *Vaccine 25*: 5086–5096, 2007.

Smith, J., et al. Cost effectiveness of a rotavirus immunization program for the United States. *Pediatrics 96*, 609–615, 1995.

Smyth, G. B., Dagley, K., and Tainsh, J. Insights into the economic consequences of the 2007 equine influenza outbreak in Australia. *Aust. Vet. J. 89*: Suppl. 1, 151–158, 2011.

Xue, Y., Kristiansen, I. S., and Freiesleben de Blasio, B. Modeling the cost of influenza: The impact of missing costs of unreported complications and sick leave. *BMC Public Health 10*: 724. http://www.biomedcentral.com/.

Hepatitis, the blood supply, noroviruses, and other endemic human pathogens

Bull, R. A., et al. Rapid evolution of pandemic noroviruses of the GII.4 lineage. *Plos Pathogens 6* (3): e1000831, 2010.

CDC Division of Viral Hepatitis. *Disease burden from viral hepatitis A, B, C in the United States.* http://www.cdc.gov/hepatitis/Statistics/2009Surveillance/index.htm.

CDC Morbidity and Mortality Weekly Report Progress Toward Strengthening National Blood Transfusion Services in 14 Countries, 2008–2010.   http://www.cdc.gov/mmwr/preview/mmwrhtml/mm6046a2.htm.

Chen, S. L., and Morgan, T. R. The natural history of hepatitis C virus (HCV) infection. *Int. J. Med Sci. 3*: 47–52, 2006.

Kaplowitz, J. G., et al. A serologic follow-up of the 1942 epidemic of postvaccination hepatitis in the United States Army. *N. Engl. J. Med. 316*: 965–970, 1987.

Measles and Rubella. 2009. WHO. http://www.euro.who.int/en/what-we-do/health topics/communicable-diseases/measles-and-rubella.

Shrestha M. P., et al. Safety and efficacy of a recombinant hepatitis E vaccine. *New. Engl. J. Med. 356*: 895–903, 2007.

Immunity, vaccines, and immune deficiency

Bolstrigdge, J., et al. Helminth therapy to treat Crohn's and other auto-immune diseases. *Parasitology Research Monograph 1*: 211–225, 2011.

Dean, A. S., et al. Incompletely matched influenza vaccine still provides protection in frail elderly. *Vaccine 28*: 864–886, 2010.

Falsey, A. R., and Walsh, E. E. Respiratory syncytial virus infection in elderly adults. *Drugs & Aging 22*: 577–587, 2005.

Kotturi, M. F., et al. A multivalent and cross-protective vaccine strategy against arenaviruses associated with human disease. *PloS Pathogens 5*: e1000695, 2009.

Kupferschmidt, K. 2011. Taking a new shot at a TB vaccine. *Science 334*: 1488–1490, 2011.

Openshaw, P. J. M., and Dunning, J. Influenza vaccination: Lessons learned from the pandemic (H1N1) 2009 influenza outbreak. *Mucosal Immunology 3*: 422–424, 2010.

Warfield, K. L., and Aman, M. J. Advances in virus-like particle vaccines for filoviruses. *J. Infect. Dis 204*: Supplement 3: S1053–S1059, 2011.

Influenza

Bokalow, S., et al. Severe H1N1-infection during pregnancy. *Arch. Gynecol. Obstet. 284*: 1133–1135, 2012.

Brody, H., et al. Influenza. *Nature 480* (7376) S1–s15, 2011.

Brundage, J. F., and Shanks, G. D. Deaths from bacterial pneumonia during the 1918–19 influenza pandemic. *Emerg. Infect. Dis. 14*: 1193–1199. 2008.

Cunha, P. A. Influenza: Historical aspects of epidemics and pandemics. *Infect. Dis. Clin. N. Am. 18*: 141–155, 2004.

Dunning, J., and Openshaw, P. J. M. Impact of the 2009 influenza pandemic. *Thorax 65*: 471–472, 2010.

Flint, S. M., et al. Disproportionate impact of pandemic (H1N1) 2009 influenza on indigenous people in the top end of Australia's Northern Territory. *Med. J. Aust 192*: 617–622, 2010.

Hung, L. S. R. The SARS epidemic in Hong Kong: What lessons have we learned? *J. Roy. Soc. Med. 96*: 374–378, 2003.

La Ruche, M., et al. The 2009 pandemic H1N1 influenza and indigenous populations of the Americas and the Pacific. *Eurosurveillance 14*: 51–56, 2009.

Michaan, N., et al. Maternal and neonatal outcome of pregnant women infected with H1N1 influenza virus (swine flu). *J. Maternal-Fetal & Neonatal Med. 25*: 130–132, 2012.

Noah, M. A., et al. Referral to an extracorporeal membrane oxygenation center and mortality among patients with severe 2009 influenza A (H1N1). *JAMA 306*: 1659–1668, 2011.

Taubenberger, J. K., Hultin, J. V., and Morens, D. M. Discovery and characterization of the 1918 pandemic influenza virus in historical context. *Antiviral Therapy 12*: 581–591, 2007.

Webster, R. G., Bean, W. J., Gorman, O. T., Chambers, T. M., and Kawaoka, Y. Evolution and ecology of influenza A viruses. *Microbiol. Rev. 56*: 152–179, 1992.

Yuen, K. Y., Peiris, M., et al. Clinical features and rapid viral diagnosis of human disease associated with avian influenza A H5N1 virus. *Lancet 351*: 467–471, 1998.

Mad cow disease and the spongiform encephalopathies

Armitage, W. J., Tullo, A. B., and Ironside, J. W. Risk of Creutzfeldt–Jakob disease transmission by ocular surgery and tissue transplantation. *Eye 23*: 1926–1930, 2009.

Berger, J. R., Weisman, E., and Weisman, B. Creutzfeldt-Jakob disease and eating squirrel brains. *The Lancet 350*: 642, 1997.

Forge, F., and Frechette, J. D. Mad cow disease and Canada's cattle industry. 2005.

Haley, N. J., et al. Detection of chronic wasting disease prion proteins in salivary, urinary and intestinal tissues of deer: Possible mechanisms of prion shedding and transmission. *J. Virol. 85*: 6309–6318, 2011.

Library of Parliament Information and Research Service. http://www.parl.gc.ca/Content/LOP/researchpublications/prb0301-e.htm.

Prusiner, S. B. 1997. Nobel Lecture. http://www.nobelprize.org/media-player/index.php?id=1714.

Rich, J. A., and Hall, S. M. BSE case associated with prion protein gene mutation. *PLoSPathogens 4*: e1000156, 2008.

Sigurdson, C. J., and Miller, M. W. Other animal prion diseases. *Brit. Med. Bull.66*: 199–212, 2003.

Smith, P. G., and Bradley, R. Bovine spongiform encephalopathy and its epidemiology. *Brit. Med. Bull. 66*: 185–198, 2003.

Pandemics, epidemics, and outbreaks

Bitar, D. M., Goubar, A., and Desenclos, J. C. International travels and fever screening during epidemics: A literature review on the effectiveness and potential use of non-contact infrared thermometers. *Eurosurveillance 14* (6): 1–4, 2009. www.eurosurveillance.org.

Budd, L., Bell, M. and Brown, T. Of plagues, planes and politics: Controlling the global spread of infectious diseases by air. *Political Geography 28*: 426–435, 2009.

Falsey, A. R., et al. Long-term care facilities: A cornucopia of viral pathogens. *J. Am. Geriat. Soc 56*: 1281–1285, 2008.

Foxwell, A. R., Roberts, L., Lokuge, K., and Kelly, P. M. Transmission of influenza on international flights, May 2009. *Emerg. Infect. Dis. 17*: 1188–1194, 2011.

Gostin, L. O., and Berkman, B. E. Pandemic influenza: Ethics, law, and the public's health. *Admin. Law Rev. 59*: 121–175, 2007.

Gralton, J., and McLaws, M. L. Protecting healthcare workers from pandemic influenza: N95 or surgical masks? *Crit. Care Med. 38*: 657–667, 2010.

Jones, R. M., and Adida, E. Influenza infection risk and predominant exposure routeuncertainty analysis. *Risk Analysis 31*: 1622–1631, 2011.

MacNeil, A., et al. Filovirus outbreak detection and surveillance: Lessons from Bundibugyo. *J. Infect. Dis. 204*: Supplement 3: S761–S767, 2011.

Morawska, L., et al. Modality of human expired aerosol size distributions. *J. Aerosol, Sci. 42*: 839–851, 2011.

Nicas, M., and Jones, R. M. Relative contributions of four exposure pathways to influenza infection risk. *Risk Analysis 29*: 1292–1303, 2009.

Osterholm, M. T. Preparing for the next pandemic *New Engl. J. Med. 352*: 1839–1842, 2005.

Pedrosa, P. B. S., and Cardosa, T. Viral infections in workers in hospital and research laboratory settings: A comparative review of infection modes and respective biosafety aspects. *Int. J. Infect. Dis.*: E366–E376, 2011.

Reissman, D. B. Pandemic influenza preparedness: Adaptive responses to an evolving challenge. *Journal of Homeland Security and Emergency Management 3* (13): June 2006. http://www.bepress.com/jhsem/vol3/iss2/13.

Suk, J. E., and Semenza, J. C. Future infectious disease threats to Europe. *Am. J. Pub. Hlth. 101*: 2068–2079, 2011.

Truscott, J., et al. Essential epidemiological mechanisms underpinning the transmission dynamics of seasonal influenza. *J. R. Soc. Interface 9*: 304–312, 2012.

SARS

Chang, K. O. Control of severe acute respiratory syndrome Singapore. *Env. Health Prevent. Med. 10*: 225–220, 2005.

Goh, K-T. Epidemiology and control of SARS in Singapore. *Ann. Acad. Med. Singapore 35*: 301–316, 2006.

Gu, J., et al. Multiple organ infection and the pathogenesis of SARS. *J. Exp. Med. 202*: 415–424, 2005.

Small, M., Tse, T. K. and Walker, D. M. Super-spreaders and the rate of transmission of the SARS virus. *Physica. D. 215*: 146–158, 2006.

INDEX

Africa
  Chikungunya virus in, 110
  dengue epidemics in, 109
  Ebola in, 95
  HIV/AIDS in, 126, 129–131
  Kaposi's sarcoma virus in, 132
  Lassa fever arenavirus in, 100
  skin infection in, 69–70
  travel to, 179
  yellow fever virus in, 106
African filoviruses, 92
agar plates, 7–8
AIDS *see* HIV/AIDS
algae, 9
Alibeck, Ken, 171
Allen, Woody, 191
Alpers, Michael, 145
Alzheimer's disease, 51
American Red Cross/Harvard
  Hospital, 18
*America's Forgotten Pandemic: The
  Influenza of 1918* (Crosby),
  xxviii
amphibians and reptiles, 167
*And the Band Played on: Politics,
  People, and the AIDS Pandemic*
  (Shilts), xxxiv
Andrewes, Christopher, 18, 80
animals and infection

antibiotics in animal feed, 68
antigenic drift and shift, xxvf,
  72, 74–78, 75f, 77f
avoiding infection, 101
cats, 53, 166–167
cattle disease, 66, 155–156
chickens, 29, 53, 59, 117
civet cats, 59–60, 61
Ebola, 94–96
ferrets, 80, 81
filoviruses, 92
hemorrhagic disease, 96–101
henipaviruses, 92–94
horses, 93, 94, 110, 163
human and animal interaction,
  166–168
human vs. animal pandemics,
  165–166
imported animals, 166–168
mouse hepatitis virus, 59
primates, 20, 29, 129–130
rabbits, 115, 158–162
rabies and related lyssaviruses,
  90–92
rodents, 50, 99–100
see also bats; birds; infection and
  immunity; mad cow disease
  and vCJD; pigs; sheep
animal virology, 14

anthrax, 7, 171, 175–177
antibiotics
    animal feed, 68
    bacterial diseases/infections,
        15–17, 117
    hemorrhagic disease, 96
    tuberculosis, 67, 70, 97
antibodies, monoclonal, 37–39
antibody tests, 10
antiviral drugs, 16, 73, 181
arbovirus *see* virus vectors
Argentina, 102, 157
Armand, Paul, 161
Armed Forces Institute
    for Medical Research
    (AFRIMS), 176
Asia
    arboviruses in, 105, 106
    Chikungunya virus in, 112
    dengue epidemics in, 109
    influenza A viruses in, 82
    SARS outbreak and exotic
        species in, 59–60
    travel to, 181
    see also Pacific countries
Asian Pacific Biosafety
    Association (APBSA), 61
Austin, Thomas, 159
Australia
    abalone infectious outbreak
        in, 164
    deliberate introduction of an
        animal virus in, 158–162
    epidemic polyarthritis with
        rash in, 110
    equine influenza in, 163
    H_5N_1 virus in, 163
    Hendra virus in, 93, 94
    HIV/AIDS in, 128
    indigenous peoples, 162
    influenza vaccines in, 84–85
    insect-born viruses in, 102, 105
    Lyme disease in, 111
    lyssaviruses in, 91
    rabbits in, 115, 158–162
    rabies, 91

bacterial infections and
    antibiotics, 117
bacterium
    bacterial disease treatment,
        15–17, 117
    flesh eating, 68
    size, 13–15
    size of, 13–15
    virus vs., 2–9
Baltimore, David, 11
Bangladesh, Nipah virus, 93
Barmah Forest virus, 112
Barré-Sinoussi, Françoise, 136
Barry, John, xxvi, xxviii, xxix
bats
    henipaviruses, 94
    hosts of viruses that infect
        humans, 92–93
    rabies, 90–91
    SARS, 61, 90
B cell and T cell receptor (TCR)
    repertoires, 32–37, 38–39
Beijerinck, Martinius, 13
Bernard, Claude, 22
Bernard Nocht Institute
    (Hamburg), 59
Bill and Melinda Gates
    Foundation, 70
biological warfare during World
    War II, 50
Biosafety Level (BSL) 1 to 4,
    20–21
bioterrorism
    anthrax, 175–177
    Hussein and WMD, 171
    novel bioterror scenarios,
        177–178
    pandemics caused by terrorists,
        169–171, 178
    rogue states, 171–173
    smallpox, 173–175

birds
  chickens, 29, 53, 59, 117
  fever and, 78
  H$_5$N$_1$ avian influenza, 19
  importation of, 167
  influenza A viruses, xxv*f*, 75–76,
    75*f*, 77*f*, 78–79, 82
  louping ill, 105
  Marek's disease, 29
  TB, 69
  West Nile virus, 103, 104
Blewett, Neal, 128
blood donation and West Nile
    virus, 103
blood transfusions, 121,
    123–124, 136
Blumberg, Baruch, 109
body orifices, 22
bone meal, 148
Boremann, Marie Luise, xxxi
bovine TB, 69
Boylston, Zabdiel, 6
Brazil, dengue and yellow fever
    outbreaks, 102
breast milk, 27
British Medical Research Council
    (MRC) Common Cold Unit
    (CCU), 18, 80
Bronz Zoo (new York), 103
Bulgaria, foot and mouth
    disease in, 157
Burkitt's lymphoma, 132–133
Burmese pythons, 164
Burnet, Macfarlane, 160
Buruli (Bairnsdale, Kumusi)
    ulcers, 69–70
Bush, George W., 127
bush meat, 130

California, West Nile virus,
    103, 104
Canada
  British beef and cattle
    imports, 149
  malaria in, 111
  SARS in, 152, 155
  transmissible spongiform
    encephalopathy in, 150
  vCJD in, 143, 148
  West Nile virus in, 103
  see also North America
cancer
  Epstein Barr virus, 29
  HIV/AIDS and, 132–133
  immunosuppression from
    treatment for, 29
  RNA tumor viruses, 11–12
cannibalism, 145
Caribbean, dengue virus in the,
    106
cats, 53, 166–167
cattle disease, 66, 155–156
  see also mad cow disease and
    vCJD
Centers for Disease Control
    (CDC)
  on bioterrorism, 170
  on economic costs from
    influenza, 152
  responsibilities during
    outbreaks, 185
  on West Nile Virus, 103, 112
  world health and the, 127
chicken pox, 29, 117
chickens, 29, 53, 59
Chikungunya virus, 110, 112
children and infants
  aspirin and, 188
  childhood illnesses, 117
  cleanliness and, 191
  dehydration in, 117
  HIV/AIDS, 127
  as multipliers of infection, 194
  vaccines, 41, 88–89, 191
  virus diarrheas, 115–116
Children's Crusade of 1212, 51
China
  hepatitis vaccine in, 120

China (*Cont.*)
  practice of variolation, 5–6
  SARS, 57, 60, 62, 63
cholera, 15, 117
Chopin, Frederic, 67
chronic obstructive pulmonary
  disease (COPD), 51
Churchill, Randolph, 15
civet cats, 59–60, 61
climate change, 9, 177
colds and minor/seasonal flu,
  17–19, 57, 59, 71–72, 74
cold sores, 29
Cold War, 170
Common Cold Unit (CCU), 18, 80
commensal microorganisms, 28
Contagion (2011), xxxii, 20, 48, 94
Conviction (2010), 11
COPD (chronic obstructive
  pulmonary disease), 51
Cornwell, Patricia, 20
coronaviruses (CoVs) pathogens,
  59, 61
cough etiquette, 24, 25, 184, 189,
  194, 198
cowpox virus, 22
cows *see* cattle disease; mad cow
  disease and vCJD
Creutzfeldt-Jakob disease *see* mad
  cow disease and vCJD
Crichton, Michael, xxiv
Crohn's disease, 191
Crosby, Alfred, xxviii
CSI, 20
cytomegalovirus (CMV), 29

Dancing Naked in the Mind Field
  (Mullis), 11
Daschle, Tom, 175
Daughters of Mars, The
  (Keneally), xxvii
DDT, 112–113
death (mortality)
  AIDS, 127, 130, 132

animal handlers and scientists,
  29, 78, 93
bunyavirus, 100
childhood vaccination vs., 41
diphtheria, 5
food poisoning, 7
foot and mouth disease, 156
hantavirus, 99
hepatitis, 120
influenza, 57, 152
  1918–1919 pandemic,
    xxvii, xxix
  pandemics and, xxvii, 42, 48,
    130, 197
pestilence, 50
pied piper story, 51
rabies in the, 92
rotavirus, 116
SARS, 57, 64
traffic accidents, 64
tuberculosis, 67
West Nile Virus, 103, 104
yellow fever virus, 106, 109
dehydration, 116–117
dengue hemorrhagic fever
  (DHF), 106
dengue viruses, 54, 102, 106, 109
developing world, HIV/AIDS, 69,
  127–128, 139
diabetes, 51
diarrhea
  bacterial, 15
  fatal, 28
  mucus-laden fecal content, 26
  oral rehydration kits and, 188
  travelers and, 180
  viruses, 114–117
  see also gastrointestinal
    (GI) tract
diphtheria, 5
diseases, causes of, 22–26
DNA
  herpesviruses, 29
  protists/protozoa, 9

RNA vs., 9–13
    viruses, 9–13
dogs, 53, 91–92, 166–167
Down, John Langdon, xxiii
Down syndrome, xxii–xxiii
ducks, 53
Durer, Albrecht, 50
Dutch Elm disease, 55
dysentery, 26

Ebola, 20, 92, 94–96
    see also hemorrhagic disease
economic factors of infections and
        diseases
    deliberate introduction of an
        animal virus, 158–162
    emergency costs, 154–155
    foot and mouth disease,
        156–158
    influenza, 155
    regulations regarding quaran-
        tines, 168
    SARS, 152
    travel, 154–155, 164
    types and costs of infectious
        threats, 153–154
    veterinary pandemics, 162–165
Egypt, hepatitis in, 121
elderly persons
    dehydration, 117
    influenza prevention, 88, 89
    lethal influenza pneumonia, 71
    SARS, 56
    shingles, 29, 117
    travel, 180
elephantiasis, 22
encephalitis, 118
endemic infections, 54–55
Enders, John, 109
epidemic polyarthritis with
        rash, 109
epidemics see pandemics,
        epidemics, and outbreaks
epizootic, 53–54

Epstein Barr virus (EBV),
    29, 132
equine see horses
eukaryotes, 9
Europe
    agricultural subsidies, 52
    biological control of rabbits
        in, 161
    blood transfusions in, 136
    British beef and cattle
        imports, 149
    Chikungunya virus in, 112
    rabies in, 91
    TB epidemic, 67
    tick-borne viruses in, 105
    Weil's disease in, 98
    see also Specific countries
Everglades (Florida), 164
exotic pets, 164
extreme drug-resistant (XDR)
    TB, 70
eye rubbing, 116, 194

face masks, xxiii, xxvii, 62, 124,
    152, 189–190
FBI anthrax investigation, 176
feces, dog, 53
feces, viruses in ingested food,
    29–30
female reproductive tract, 22,
    23, 29
Fenner, Frank, 160
ferrets, 80, 81
fever
    birds and, 78
    children and, 117
    foot and mouth disease, 156
    infection and, 31–32
    malaria and, 183
    non-specific, 60
    pregnant women and, 168
    respiratory symptoms
        with a, 89
    ticks and, 111

fever (*Cont.*)
   travel and, 71, 117
   vaccination and, 41, 85
   see also Specific fever diseases
Finlay, Carlos, 107
Fitzgerald, Grace, xxxi
flaviviruses, 105–106
flesh-eating bacteria, 68
foot and mouth disease (FMD),
   156–158
Fore people of Papua New
   Guinea, 145
forest and wetlands habitats
   destruction, 70, 196
Four Horsemen of the Apocalypse
   (Durer), 50
France, 149, 161
frogs, 164

Gadjusek, Carleton, 145
gangrene and trench foot, 54–55
gastrointestinal (GI) tract, 22,
   23–24, 28, 29–30
   ecomomic factors, 153–154
   intussusception, 116
   see also diarrhea; pathogens,
     single-host human
Gates, Bill, 127
GAVI initiative, 185
gay-related immunodeficiency
   disease (GRID), 135
German measles (rubella),
   27, 117
Germany, Marburg virus, 95
Gibbs, Joe, 145
GI tract *see* gastrointestinal
   (GI) tract
Given Day, The (Lehane), xxvii
Global Fund to Fight AIDS,
   Tuberculosis and Malaria, 127
Global Program on AIDS, 49
Gorgas, William, 107
Great Influenza, The (Barry), xxvi,
   xxviii, xxix

GRID (gay-related
   immunodeficiency
   disease), 135
Griffin, Elizabeth, 29

H_1N_1
   classification of, 48
   economic factors, 152–153
   influenza of 2009, 77f
   mild nature of, 43–44, 44–45
   1918–1919 pandemic flu virus,
     79–81, 80
   pediatric deaths, 85
   vaccine, xxiii–xxiv, 84
   see also pandemic flu virus of
     1918–1919
H_2N_2 Asian pandemic (1957), 82
H_3N_2 Hong Kong pandemic
   (1968), 74–75, 75f, 82
H_3N_8 influenza A virus, 168
H_5N_1 avian influenza (AI) viruses
   classification of, 48
   HPAI (hi-path) and LPAI
     (lo-path), 19
   Level 6 pandemic, 162
   priority for surveillance, 82
   spread between humans, 78
   transmission of, 81
   zoonotic transmission, 53
H7N9, xxxviii, 76
HAART (highly active anti-
   retroviral therapy), 136–137,
   139, 140, 141, 142
hand hygiene, 23, 24, 116, 184,
   189, 194
hantaviruses, 99
Harris, Charles Stuart, 80
hemorrhagic disease, 20, 92,
   94–101, 105, 106
Hendra virus, 93
henipaviruses, 92–94
hepatitis
   antiviral drugs, 16
   A virus, 26, 119

blood transfusions and, 123, 124
B virus, 61, 109, 121–122
chronic hepatitis dangers,
    122–123
C virus, 16, 27, 54, 121–122,
    125, 194
vaccine, 119–121
Herpes simplex (HSV), 29
herpesviruses, 29
Hesse, Fanny, 8
Hiddel, Marie Louise, xxxi
highly active anti-retroviral
    therapy *see* HAART
Hindenburg, Paul von, xxvi
Hitler, Adolf, 178
HIV/AIDS
    attention received initially, 194
    blood transfusions and, 123, 124
    changes to virus, 138–139
    classification of, 48
    curing, 139–142
    current situation for, 126–129
    endemic infection, 54
    HAART, 136–137, 139, 140,
        141, 142
    HIV developing into AIDS,
        36–37
    immune system and,
        29, 131–133
    measles and, 118
    origins of, 129–131
    overview, 142
    progress regarding, 136–138
    retrovirus, 11
    science and, 135–136
    tests for, 37
    transmission of, 27
    treatments, 16–17
    tuberculosis and, 67, 69
    vaccine, 86, 133–135, 173
Hong Kong, SARS, 57, 60
Hong Kong flu (1968), 53
horizontal infections, 26–27
horses

equine encephalitis viruses, 110
Hendra virus, 94
henipaviruses, 93
racehorses and influenza
    outbreaks, 163
Hultin, Johan, 80
human papilloma virus, 109
human population, 198
Hussein, Saddam, 171
hydatid disease, 53
hypodermic needles, 23, 27

immunity *see* infection and
    immunity
India, 50, 105
indigenous peoples, 162
Indonesia, Chikungunya virus
    in, 110
infants *see* children and infants
infection and immunity
    bacterial and viral disease
        treatment, 15–17
    causes of disease, 22–26
    cleanliness and, 190–191
    endemic infection, 54–55
    herd immunity, 125, 180
    horizontal infection, 26–27
    immune response, 31–37
    immune system evolution,
        30–31
    immunity defined, 30
    laboratories and infection, 61
    monoclonal antibodies, 37–39
    non-harmful microorganisms,
        27–28
    pandemics and infection,
        51–52
    passive immunization, 7
    pathogens, 19–21
    public misunderstanding, 1–2
    RNA and DNA, 9–13
    vaccines, 40–41
    vertical transmission, 27
    virome, 28–30

infection and immunity (*Cont.*)
   virus and bacterium size,
      13–15
   virus vs. bacterium, 2–9
   see also animals and infection
infectious bronchitis virus, 59
influenza
   A and B viruses, 40, 72, 72–74,
      74, 82
   antigenic drift and shift, xxv*f*,
      72, 74–78, 75*f*, 77*f*
   anti-influenza drugs, 16, 73,
      86–87
   A virus particles, 3*f*
   capacity to counter, 82–83
   colds and minor flu, 17–19, 59
   C virus, 72
   fear of, 88–89
   high-path infections, 19
   horizontal infections, 26
   immune-escape variant, 49
   immunity, xxiv
   kinds of influenza viruses,
      72–74
   lo-path infections, 19
   old and very dangerous nature
      of, 66
   Pandemic Alert Phase, 45,
      46*f*, 47
   as pandemic threat, 70–72
   prevention apart from vaccines,
      16, 73, 86–88
   seasonal, 57, 71–72, 74
   vaccine, 14
   vaccine research and
      production, 83–86
   see also economic factors for
      infections and disease;
      Specific influenza viruses
influenza pandemic of 2009, 25,
      50, 77*f*
insect-borne infection *see*
      mosquito/insect-borne
      infections

Institut Pasteur, Rue du Docteur
      Roux (Paris, France), 8
International Convention on
      the Prohibition of the
      Development, Production
      and Stockpiling of
      Bacteriological (Biological)
      and Toxin Weapons and on
      their Destruction, 170–171
Internet, 52
intussusception, 116
Iran Jaya (West Papua),
      Chikungunya virus, 110
Iraq, 171
Ivins, Bruce, 176–177

Japan, 143, 157
Japanese encephalitis virus (JEV),
      105, 112
Jenner, Edward, 5, 6, 22, 23
Jerne, Nils, 38
Jurassic Park (Crichton), xxiv

Kaposi's sarcoma virus
      (KSHV), 132
Keats, John, 67
Keneally, Tom, xxvii
Kennedy, John F., 106
Koch, Robert, xxv, 8, 67, 80
Kohler, Georges, 38
Korea, foot and mouth disease
      in, 157
Krafft, Amy, 80
Kunjin virus, 105
Kyasanur Forest disease, 105

laboratories and infection, 61
Langerhan's cells, 22
Lassa fever arenavirus, 100
Leahy, Patrick, 175
Lehane, Dennis, xxvii
leprosy, 15
Lesseps, Ferdinand de, 107
Lipkin, Ian, xxxii

Lyme disease, 111
lymphatic system, 22–23
lymphocytic choriomeningitis
   virus, 61

mAb technology, 37–39
MacNamara, Jean, 159–160
mad cow disease and vCJD
   bone meal, 148
   British meats and cattle
      importation, 148–149
   overview, 143–144
   pandemic risk, 149, 150–151
   transmissible spongiform
      encephalopathy, 144–146,
      149–150
malaria, 1, 9, 111, 127, 132, 183
Malaysia, 93, 110
Mallon, Mary, 68
Marburg virus, 92, 95–96
Marek's disease, 29
masks *see* face masks
Mather, Cotton, 6
Mathews, John, 145
measles, 27, 117, 118–119, 185
media, on food poisoning, 7
Medical Research Council
      Laboratories at Mill Hill, 80
Mein Kampf (Hitler), 177
meningoencephalitis, 104
Mexico, 103
   see also North America
mice and infections, 99–100
microbiology, history of, 8
Middle East, bat coronavirus in, 61
milk, pasteurizing, 67
Milstein, Cesar, 38
Minerva, 30
MMR vaccine, 117
monoclonal antibodies, 37–39
mortality *see* death (mortality)
mosquito/insect-borne infections,
      23, 54, 100–101, 105, 110–111,
      180–181

see also Specific diseases; virus
   vectors
mouse hepatitis virus, 59
Mullis, Kary, 11
multi-drug-resistant (MDR)
   typhoid, 68
multi-drug-resistant TB, 68–70
Murphy, Lillian, xxxi
Murray Valley encephalitis
   virus, 105

National Institutes of Health
   (NIH), 127
National University Hospital
   (Singapore), 58
Navajo flu, 99
necrotizing fasciolitis, 68
needles, hypodermic, 23, 27
needles, tattoo, 181–182
neuraminidase inhibitors, 17
New Zealand, 161, 162
Nigeria, murders of health care
   workers in, 169
1918–1919 pandemic flu *see*
   pandemic flu virus of
   1918–1919
Nipah virus, 93
Nobel Prize, 8, 11, 33, 38, 109, 140,
   145, 147
noroviruses, 114–115
North America
   British beef and cattle
      imports, 149
   dengue epidemics in, 109
   indigenous peoples, 162
   rabies in, 91
   tick-borne viruses in, 105
   transmissible spongiform
      encephalopathy in, 149–150
   yellow fever in, 109
   see also Specfic countries
nose picking, 24, 63, 116, 194
nosocomial spread, 58
nuclear weapons, 172

obesity, 51
OIE (Organization Internationale des Epizootiques), 53
Outbreak (1995), xxxii
outbreaks *see* pandemics, epidemics, and outbreaks

Pacific countries
  arboviruses in, 105, 106
  dengue epidemics in, 109
  indigenous peoples, 162
  skin infection in, 69–70
  see also Asia
Pakistan, murders of health care workers in, 169
Pale Horse, Pale Rider (Porter), xxvii
Panama Canal, 107
pandemic flu virus of 1918–1919
  classification of, 48
  H_1N_1 serotype, 35–36
  research regarding, 79–81
  vs. terrorism, 185–186
  worldwide spead, 42
pandemics, epidemics, and outbreaks
  animal vs. human, 165–166
  BSE/vCJD, 149
  different characteristics of, 49–51, 55
  endemic infections, 54–55
  foot and mouth disease, 157–158
  infection and pandemics, 51–52
  overview, 195–199
  pandemic classification system, refining, 48–49
  pandemic classification system (current), 45–47, 46f
  pandemic defined, 42–43
  panics and, xxi
  plant pandemics, 55
  rich vs. poor countries, 47
  vectored viruses, 111–113
  veterinary, 162–165
  WHO declaration of pandemics, 43–44
  WHO operations, 45–47, 46f
  widespread infections and pandemics, 114
  zoonosis, 52–54
pandemics, protecting humanity from and during
  cleanliness, 190–192
  family protection, 187–190
  individuals' actions, 179–182, 184–186
  local community involvement, 186–187
  overview, 193–194
  seeking help during a pandemic, 192–193
  symptoms of infection, 182–184
  while traveling, 182
panzootic, 53–54
Papua New Guinea, 145
Paraguay, dengue and yellow fever outbreaks, 102
Pasteur, Louis, xxv, 8, 91, 92
pasteurizing milk, 67
pathogens, single-host human
  blood transfusions, 121, 123–124
  hepatitis, 119–123
  intussusception, 116
  measles, 118–119
  pandemics caused by, 124–125
  protecting against GI tract infections, 116
  skin spots, 117
  virus diarrheas, 114–117
  widespread infections and pandemics, 114
pathogens overview, 19–21
PCR *see* polymerase chain reaction
Peace Corp, 106

pestilence, 50
Peterson, Robert, 154
Petri, Julius, 7
Petri plates, 7–8
pets, exotic, 164
Philippines, 95
Phipps, James, 22
phlegm and snot, 23, 26, 88
Pied Piper of Hamelin, 50–51
pigs
    FMD virus, 155, 158
    henipaviruses, 93–94
    Hong Kong flu (1968), 53
    influenza A viruses, xxvf, 49,
        75f, 76–77, 77f, 82
    influenza C virus strain, 72
    influenza transmitted between,
        79–80
    Japanese B encephalitis
        virus, 105
Place, Edna, xxxi
plague
    defined, 50
    in medieval Europe, 48,
        50, 193
    use of the term, 50–51
plant pandemics, 55
pneumonia, laboratory
    research, 80
"The Poetry of Sleazy Songs
    and Rotten Rhymes"
    (website), 23
polio, 15, 40, 109, 118, 185
politics
    bioterrorism and, 170
    evidence-based and
        pragmatic, 129
    extremist political agendas and
        rhetoric, 177, 188
    health of citizens and, 170
    importation and local
        producers, 157
    narrow parochialism, 177
    public health and, 185, 198

    see also public officials and
        politicians
polymerase chain reaction (PCR),
    11–12, 17, 59, 64
Porter, Katharine Anne, xxvii
pregnant women see women,
    pregnant
primates, 20, 29, 129–130
protists/protozoa, 9
protozoan malaria parasite, 107
public health measures/services
    bacterial and viral diseases,
        15–16
    bioterrorism and, 186
    evidence-based and pragmatic,
        129, 194
    information during an out-
        break, 188, 192, 193
    knowledge and, 82
    maintaining investment in, 65
    rabies and, 91
    smallpox and, 174
    state and local, 186
    support/funding for, xxxiii, 63,
        65, 184, 198
public officials and politicians
    harm-reduction strategies,
        xxxiv
    HIV/AIDS and, 128, 135
    pandemic of 1918–1919, xxvii
    vaccines and national
        defense, 189
    see also politics
pulmonary syndrome, 99

rabbit calicivirus, 115
rabbits in Australia, 158–162
rabies, 90–92
Reed, Walter, 107
Reich, Kathy, 20
Reid, Ann, 80
Relenza, 17, 73, 86–87, 181
reproductive tract infections,
    22, 23, 29

Republic of the Congo, Ebola, 95
respiratory syncytial virus
    (RSV), 88
respiratory tract, 22, 23,
    23–26, 28
    see also influenza; SARS (severe
    acute respiratory syndrome);
    tuberculosis (TB)
retrovirus
retrovirus, 11–12
rhinoviruses, 17–18
Rift Valley Fever Virus
    bunyavirus, 100
RNA, DNA vs., 9–13
Robbins, Fred, 109
Rockefeller Institute, 109
Rockwell, Sam, 11
rodents, 50, 99–100
rodents and infections, 99–100
rotavirus, 26
Roux, Emil, 91
rubella (German measles), 27, 117
Russia, 105, 170
Ruth, Babe, xxvii

Sabin, Albert, 15
    see also polio vaccine
Salk, Jonas, 15
SARS (severe acute respiratory
    syndrome)
    bats as carriers, 90
    causes of, 59–61
    economic impact of, xxiii,
        152, 155
    long-term effects and lessons
        learned, 63–65
    potential sources for, 61
    scary nature of, 56–57
    spread of, 49–50, 57–58
    steps taken to stop the
        outbreak, 61–63
Saudi Arabia, vCJD in, 148
Scandinavia, scrapie in, 144
scarlet fever (Streptococcus), 117

Scotland, 91, 144, 156
scrapie, 144–145, 147–148
serotypes, 12
severe acute respiratory syn-
    drome see SARS
sexual activity, 181
sheep
    FMD virus, 156
    scrapie, 144–145, 147–148
    tapeworm, 53
    tick-borne viruses, 105
Shilts, Randy, xxxiv
shingles, 29, 117
Shope, Richard E., 79, 159
Silent Witness, 20
Singapore General, 58
Singapore SARS outbreak, 57–58,
    60, 62, 64, 152
single-host human pathogens
    see pathogens, single-host
    human
skin and infection, 22–23
smallpox
    bioterrorism using, 172,
        173–175
    cost of eradication, 185
    vaccination, 5–6, 172, 173
Smith, Wilson, 80
snot and phlegm, 23, 26, 88
Soderbergh, Steven, xxxii
South America
    bat-rabies, 91
    dengue epidemics in, 109
    hemorrhagic fever viruses, 100
    skin infection in, 69–70
    West Nile virus in, 103, 109
    yellow fever virus in, 106, 109
    see also Specific countries
Soviet Union, 5, 171
Spanish flu see pandemic flu virus
    of 1918–1919
spongiform encephalopathy see
    mad cow disease and vCJD
Spurlock, Morgan, 51

staphylococcal scalded skin
    syndrome, 117
Stop TB Partnership, 70
subacute sclerosing
    panencephalitis (SSPE), 119
sulfonamides, 16
Supersize Me (2004), 51
Swank, Hilary, 11
swine flu *see* H₁N₁
syndrome, defined, xxii–xxiii
syphilis, 15

Tamiflu, 17, 73, 86–87, 181
Tang Tock Seng Public Hospital
    (Singapore), 57–58
Tanzania, Chikungunya virus, 110
tattoos, 181–182
Taubenberger, Jeffrey, xxiv, 80, 81
TB *see* tuberculosis
T cell receptor (TCR) repertoires,
    32–37, 38–39
Temin, Howard, 11
tetanus, 7
Thailand, 110, 135
Thatcher, Margaret, 199
Theiler, Max, 109
*Their Fate is Our Fate: How Birds
    Foretell Threats to Our Health
    and Our World (Doherty)*, 14
ticks, 105, 110–111
Time Magazine, 178
tissue culture technology, 17
Toronto, Canada, 60
toxoplasmosis, 53
travel
    economic costs of infections
        and, 154–155, 164
    influenza and, 71–72, 83
    pandemics and, 179–184, 195
    SARS and, 61, 62
    unwell passengers, 165–166
    vCJD and, 144
trench foot and gangrene, 54–55
tsetse flies, 23

tuberculosis (TB)
    blood-contaminated mucus, 97
    extreme drug-resistant
        (XDR), 70
    Global Fund to Fight
        AIDS, Tuberculosis and
        Malaria, 127
    history and current situation
        regarding, 66
    in literature, 15
    multi-drug-resistant (MDR)
        TB, 68–70
    old and very dangerous
        nature of, 66
    vaccine, 40, 67
typhoid, 68, 117
Typhoid Mary, 68
Tyrrell, David, 18

UNAIDS, 70
UN Food and Agriculture
    Organization, 53
United Kingdom
    biological weapons
        program, 170
    bioterrorism concerns in
        the, 170
    blood transfusions in the, 123
    economic impact of infections
        in the, 153–154
    FMD epidemic in the,
        156–157, 158
    influenza pandemic of
        2009, 25
    tick-borne viruses in the, 105
    vCJD in the, 143, 146, 148
United States
    agricultural subsidies, 51
    anthrax attack in the, 174–175
    biological weapons
        program, 170
    bioterrorism concerns in
        the, 170
    blood transfusions in the, 136

United States (*Cont.*)
  dengue viruses in the, 106
  Ebola, 95
  economic impact of infections
    in the, 153, 154
  equine encephalitis viruses in
    the, 110
  hantavirus in the, 99
  hepatitis in the, 121
  HIV/AIDS in the, 110–119
  indigenous peoples, 162
  Lyme disease in the, 111
  malaria in the, 111
  noroviruses in the, 115
  pediatric deaths from
    influenza, 85
  public health activities, 186
  rabies in the, 91
  seasonal influenza, 57, 72, 84
  transmissible spongiform
    encephalopathy in the, 150
  2012–2013 winter flu season,
    78, 89
  vCJD in the, 143
  West Nile virus in the, 102–104,
    109, 111–112, 154, 168
  yellow fever virus in the, 109,
    109–110
  see also North America
UN Millennium Development
  Goal 4, 185
U.S. Armed Forces Institute of
  Pathology in Washington,
  DC, 80
U.S. Army's Medical Research
  Institute for Infectious
  Disease (USAMRID), 176
U.S. Postal Service, 175
U.S. President's Emergency
  Plan for AIDS Relief
  (PEPFAR), 127
U.S. Public Health Service
  Commissioned Corps,
  184–185

vaccination/vaccines
  about, 40–41
  broad-spectrum/universal,
    85–86
  Chikungunya virus, 110
  childhood, 41
  cost-effective nature of, 185
  development of, 16
  Ebola, 95
  engineered vaccinia, 172–173
  flaviviruses, 113
  hepatitis, 109, 119–121
  herd immunity, 125, 184
  history of, 5–6
  HIV/AIDS, 86, 133–135
  human papilloma virus, 109
  influenza, 72, 79, 83–86, 88–89
  measles, 118, 119
  meningococcemia, 96
  MMR, 117
  novel infectious agents, 188–189
  opposition to vaccination, 118,
    180, 189
  pneumonia, 71
  polio, 15, 40, 109
  seasonal influenza, 57, 74
  smallpox, 5–6, 172
  travel and, 179–180
  tuberculosis, 67
  veterinary, 113
  women of childbearing age
    and, 27
  yellow fever, 109, 121
van Leeuwenhoek, Antony, 8
variolation, 5–6
Vaughan, Victor, xxvi
vCJD *see* mad cow disease and
  vCJD
von Clausewitz, Carl, xxxi
viruses
  bacterium vs., 2–9
  colds and flu, 17–19
  diagram of, 4f
  diarrhea, 114–117

flaviviruses, 105
hantaviruses, 99
henipaviruses, 92–94
noroviruses, 114–115
pandemics and, 52
RNA and DNA, 9–13
size of, 13–15
viral disease treatment, 15–17
virus vectors
aborovirus global movement,
109–110
about, 102–103
Barmah Forest virus, 112
Chikungunya virus, 110, 112
Japanese encephalitis
virus, 112
mosquitoes and ticks, 110–111
pandemic risks, 111–113
West Nile Virus, 41, 102,
102–106, 103–106, 109,
111–112, 112
yellow fever virus, 106–109,
108f, 111
von Ludendorff, Erich, xxv–xxvi

weapons of mass
destruction, 171
Weil's disease, 98
Weller, Tom, 109
West Nile virus (WNV)
animals and, 103–106,
111–112, 166
kidney disease and, 41
Kunjin virus and, 102
in the United States, 102–103,
109, 111–112, 154
wetlands and forest habitats
destruction, 70, 196
white blood cells (WBCs), 31, 32, 62

WHO (World Health
Organization) see World
Health Organization
whooping cough, 27
women, pregnant
cats and, 53
fever and, 168
H1N1 influenza A virus
and, xxiv
parvovirus B19 and, 117
women of childbearing age and
vaccination, 27
World Health Organization
(WHO)
on AIDS pandemic, 48–49
and the CDC, 185
declaration of pandemics by,
43–44
influenza surveillance efforts
by, 82
influenza vaccine decisions, 72
operations of, 45–47, 46f
pandemic definition, 51
SARS diagnostic test, 59
on smallpox, 6
tuberculosis (TB), 66–68
World War I, 54–55, 170
World War II, 170

yellow fever virus, 106–109, 108f,
111, 121
Yerkes National Primate Center
(Atlanta, Georgia), 29
Yosemite National Park, 99
Yugoslavia, Marburg virus, 95

Zigas, Vincent, 145
Zinkernagel, Rolf, 33
zur Hausen, Harald, 109